LOW-CALORIE WEIGHT LOSS COOKBOOK

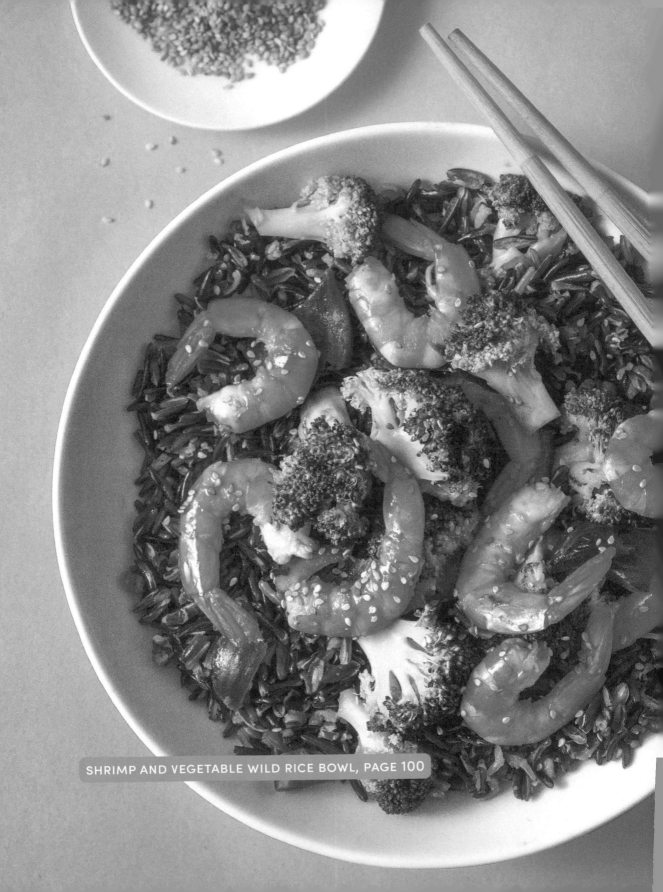

SHRIMP AND VEGETABLE WILD RICE BOWL, PAGE 100

LOW-CALORIE WEIGHT LOSS
COOKBOOK

THE 28-DAY PLAN TO TAKE CONTROL
OF YOUR HEALTH AND WEIGHT

Manuel Villacorta, MS, RDN

Photography by Annie Martin

ROCKRIDGE
PRESS

Interior and Cover Designer: Emma Hall
Art Producer: Megan Baggott
Production Editor: Mia Moran
Production Manager: Riley Hoffman

Photography © 2021 Annie Martin. Food styling by Nadine Page Beauchamp

Illustrations © 2020, 2021 Charlie Layton

Author photo courtesy of Bradford Rogne Photography

ISBN: Print 978-1-64876-665-7
eBook 978-1-64876-164-5

R0

To all of the clients I've seen in my private practice who have successfully lost weight and, most importantly, kept it off, using the lifestyle principles in this book.

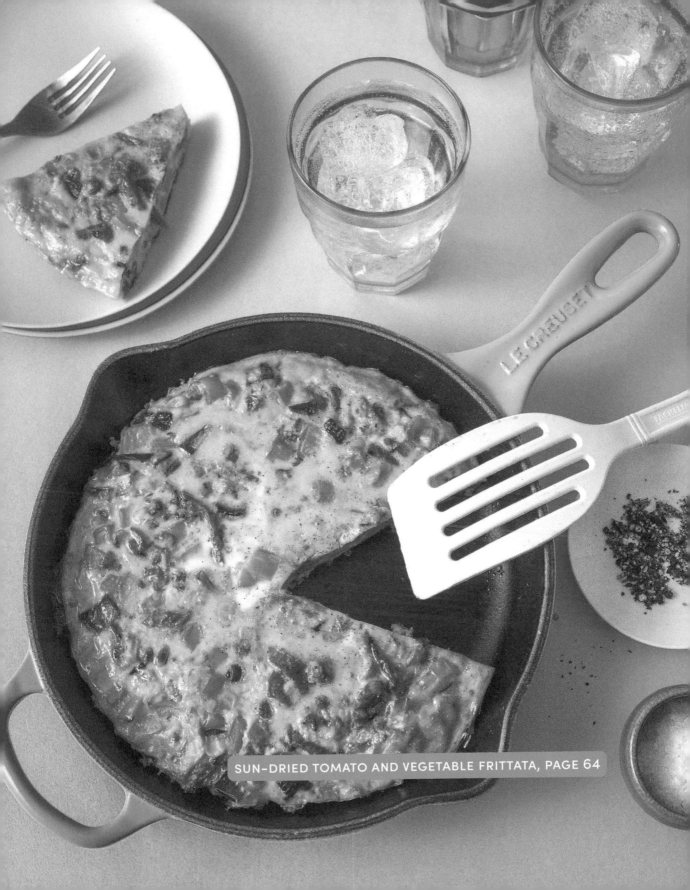

SUN-DRIED TOMATO AND VEGETABLE FRITTATA, PAGE 64

Contents

INTRODUCTION viii

Part One: Low-Calorie Living 1

CHAPTER ONE: Losing Weight 3

CHAPTER TWO: Incorporating Exercise 15

CHAPTER THREE: The Meal Plan 33

Part Two: Low-Calorie Recipes 51

CHAPTER FOUR: Breakfasts 53

CHAPTER FIVE: Lunches 77

CHAPTER SIX: Dinners 103

CHAPTER SEVEN: Snacks and Desserts 135

CHAPTER EIGHT: Kitchen Staples, Dressings, and Sauces 147

MEASUREMENT CONVERSIONS 160

RESOURCES 161

REFERENCES 162

INDEX 163

Introduction

I moved to the United States from Peru when I was barely 20 years old. With my mamá no longer cooking for me, I was forced to fend for myself in the food department. So, I did what any 20-year-old guy would do—I ate out at restaurants. However, this approach to nutrition was short-lived, as I began to notice that my wallet was getting slimmer, but my waist was not. I wrote a letter to my mother and asked her to send me my favorite recipes from home so I could cook for myself. Once I began to do this, I realized that I had a life-changing amount of control over how many calories I was eating, and how much sugar, salt, and fat were going into my food. This was my first experience recognizing the impact of low-calorie eating.

As a registered dietitian-nutritionist with 18 years of experience, and the author of five books on nutrition, weight loss, and wellness, I have helped thousands of people reach their weight loss goals. I have done this by teaching and creating programs that use a low-calorie but healthy approach to eating. When people embark on a new diet, especially a low-calorie one, they often think it has to be boring. The virtues of low-calorie eating have been diluted by unqualified individuals peddling meal plans you may be familiar with, full of bland chicken breast, steamed broccoli, and brown rice. It's often thought that the rich flavors from your favorite comfort foods are a thing of memory—and sweets? Taboo. But not this time, and not in this book. I always say that eating healthy doesn't have to be boring or daunting.

People have different motivations for changing their eating habits. Some want to lose weight, others want to learn how to control their hunger, and some just want to stay healthy. Luckily for you, this book can help you meet these goals, no matter which category you fall into. In this book, I've provided plenty of mouth-watering recipes, as well as meal plans and an exercise regimen that offers the guidance to lose weight and keep your body healthy while you do it. The meal plan is designed to give you structure, ensure you stay in your calorie range, and give you a clear road map on your road to weight loss. The exercise regimen will help supplement your low-calorie eating and play a key role in improving your health and physique.

From this book, I want you to learn how to eat low-calorie while also taking care of your health. When people pursue weight loss without guidance, they often end up just skipping random meals and eating unsatisfying "diet" foods to lose weight fast. Consequently, their health suffers. By using these recipes and meal plans to make your own meals, you can take control of your health and weight. I want this book to transcend the myths that delicious meals don't have a place in a low-calorie diet, and that to lose weight, you have to give up your favorite foods and suffer through endless bland salads. I also want to provide you with valuable tips on how to make low-calorie eating a seamless habit in your lifestyle and how to keep the weight off long after you've succeeded in reaching your goals.

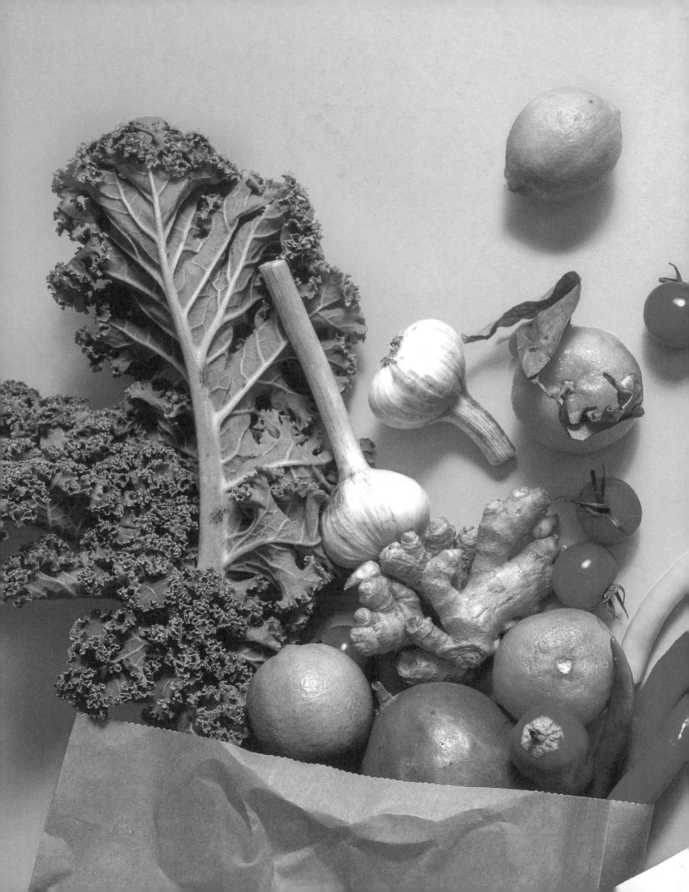

PART ONE

LOW-CALORIE LIVING

This section outlines best practices and tips for adhering to a low-calorie lifestyle, how to assess your calorie needs, and how to lose weight healthfully. You'll learn how weight loss happens, how to set achievable goals, and which foods to keep on hand to support your new way of eating. We'll explore the importance of exercise and how to execute physical activity successfully and safely. Finally, we'll walk through your low-calorie meal plan and simple guidelines for following it.

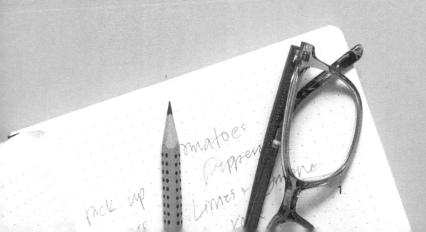

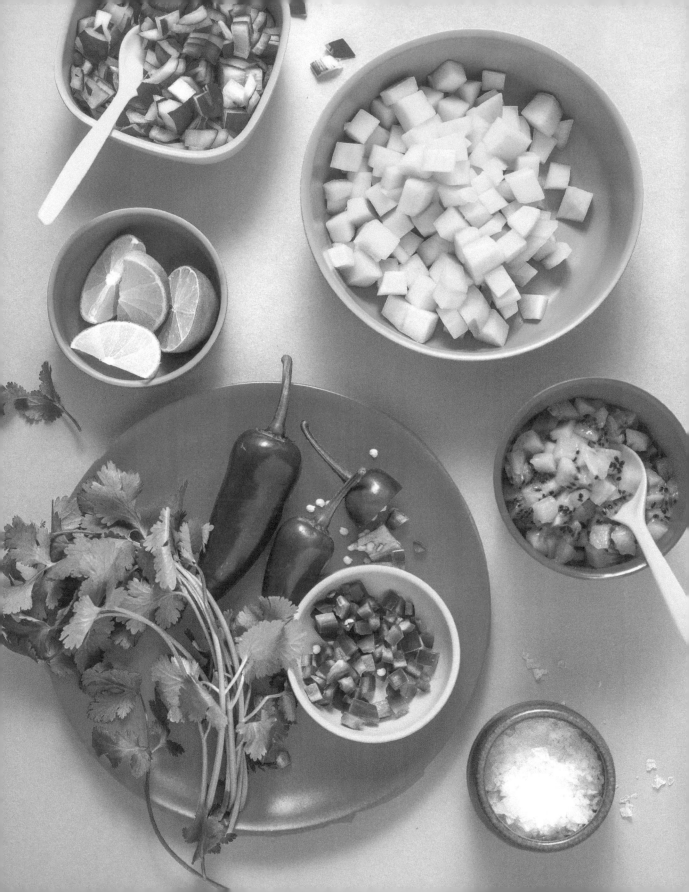

CHAPTER ONE

LOSING WEIGHT

We know we need to eat less to experience weight loss, but why? The answer: calories in, calories out. If you're taking in more calories than you are burning, you'll gain weight. If you're burning more calories than you are taking in, you'll lose weight. However, we cannot solely rely on exercise to be responsible for our "calories out." A big part of tipping that scale is adopting low-calorie eating habits so our metabolism and exercise don't have to work as hard to keep us burning. Low-calorie eating can be a scary change for some and isn't always easy, but I'll explain best practices on how to make it work for you.

The Principles of Healthy Weight Loss

Losing weight is a complex process, but not at all an impossible one. When it comes to losing and maintaining a healthy weight, "quick fixes" like fad diets or detox cleanses may give you short-term results, but they are often ineffective in the long run. More often than not, you'll gain the weight back. Why? Because they aren't sustainable, and they don't teach you anything. The goal shouldn't be to lose weight quickly, but to lose weight and keep it off in a way that's healthy for your body and mental health.

Let me be clear: Even though this is a low-calorie cookbook, I do not advocate counting calories in the long term. However, when it comes to weight loss, calories *do* matter. One piece of the weight loss equation is to eat less than what you are burning—you can't lose weight until there are fewer calories going into the body than being burned out. This is called a calorie deficit, which is the rationale for the low-calorie approach of this book. Being aware of, but not obsessing over, the portion sizes you consume (and thus the number of calories you eat), is not a form of dieting, but a lifestyle habit you can develop. This awareness will allow you to lose weight and keep it off for the long run.

You'll also want to be wary of "empty calories." A phrase you've likely heard before, "empty calories" are calories that come from food with little to no nutritional value, such as candy or alcohol. This is not to say you can't ever have candy or alcohol, but it's important to be conscious of how frequently you have them when weight loss is your goal, because they don't provide you with the nutrition needed to fuel your body, and they contribute extra calories that will slow weight loss.

LOW CALORIE, NOT STARVING

If you felt deprived while trying to lose weight in the past, you may have been taking an unnecessarily difficult approach. Eating low calorie means achieving fewer calories in than out, while still eating enough to support your health and nourish your body without over-eating. Eating too few calories can be detrimental to your health, and even to your weight loss efforts. When you eat too few calories, your body begins to become afraid that it won't have enough fuel to do its basic processes, such as keeping your heart beating and keeping you sitting upright in your desk chair. As a survival mech-anism, your body slows down its metabolism and clings to your body fat for dear life to ensure it has an energy source for later. Don't fall into this trap! Always remember that "low calorie" doesn't mean "starving."

SET SMART GOALS

Whenever my clients set goals that fail, the top reason is that their goals were either unrealistic or too broad. For example, the goal "I want to lose a lot of weight" is too broad and probably unrealistic, and without a plan, you'll probably just end up frustrated and discouraged.

To meet your health and weight loss goals, you'll want to make them SMART (specific, measurable, attainable, relevant, and time-bound). So, let's take "I want to lose a lot of weight" and turn this into a SMART goal.

- **Specific:** How much weight do you want to lose? Put a specific number on it. If you want to lose 15 pounds, make that clear.
- **Measurable:** What's your plan to track your progress? Daily weighing is not recommended, because your weight fluctuates from day to day. Instead, tell yourself you will weigh yourself weekly to monitor progress.
- **Attainable:** Make sure your goal and time line to accomplish it are within your reach. For example, even if you want to lose 50 pounds, start with 15 first. It'll be much easier and faster for you to achieve this goal, and once you do, you'll have the confidence to keep going.

- **Relevant:** What does your goal mean to you? For example, if you visited your doctor and were told that your heart health is in danger, that's a powerful motivator to remind yourself of as you work toward your goal.
- **Time-bound:** What's your time limit? Trying to lose 15 pounds over the course of 4 weeks isn't an effective goal. Give yourself a realistic time limit, such as 4 months, to achieve this goal so you don't end up disappointed.

If you have underlying health conditions such as a history or family history of disordered eating, are pregnant, or have any other potentially relevant concern, always consult with your doctor before starting any new diet or exercise regimen.

Finally, even with solid goals in place, in order to see weight loss, it's necessary to tailor mindful habits. This includes taking time to food shop, meal prep, and meal plan. This book will help make all of this far less overwhelming by providing you with delicious recipes, shopping lists, and meal plans.

EAT NUTRIENT-DENSE FOODS

Nutrient-dense foods pack in a lot of nutrition for the number of calories they deliver. For example, two apples add up to about 200 calories. A can of soda is also about 200 calories. What's the difference if all that matters is calories in versus calories out? Well, apples are nutrient-dense. Even though they have the same calorie count as soda, they are dense with fiber, vitamin C, potassium, and antioxidants, which assist the body in digestion, body tissue repair, fluid balance, immune function, and even disease prevention, while soda delivers no nutrients.

This is why a calorie is not just a calorie. The source of your calories matters, especially because you will be eating fewer calories to lose weight, so you want to make sure the calories you *are* consuming are helping nourish your body and maintain your health. Ideally, you'll want each of your meals to contain one of the "big four"—protein, produce, fat, and whole grains.

- **Protein:** Of all the macronutrients, protein will keep you feeling fuller for longer, thus controlling your hunger (key to eating low calorie). Shoot for at least 20 grams of protein in each meal.
- **Produce:** Fruits and/or vegetables, whether fresh, frozen, dried, or canned, should fill at least half of your plate for each meal.
- **Fat:** There's no specific amount recommended for fat in each meal, as it always seems to sneak its way in. However, try to make sure you are consuming healthy fats in place of saturated or trans fats when possible. These

healthy fats can come in the form of avocado, canola oil, olive oil, nuts, nut butters, and seeds.

- **Whole grains:** Whole grains such as brown rice, whole wheat bread, and quinoa are more nutritious than their whiter counterparts, and they pack more fiber to keep you full. Aim to make at least half of your grains whole, and include at least one ½ cup serving in your meals.

BE MINDFUL OF PORTION SIZES

Even if you are eating nutrient-dense foods, portion sizes matter. You could applaud yourself for eating avocado toast with an egg on whole-grain bread, but if you're eating too much of this nutritious food, weight loss will become more difficult. One way to control this is to watch your portion sizes.

Recommended portions vary depending on your sex, body size, and specific needs. However, you can use the "Talk to Your Hand" rule to figure out your serving sizes. Use your hand as a measuring tool if you're unsure of how to portion your food:

Fist (1 cup): Your fist illustrates two servings of cooked pasta, rice, or other grain.

Palm (3 to 6 ounces): Your palm is one serving of meat. Small palms measure 3 to 4 ounces and bigger palms 5 to 6 ounces.

Thumb (1 teaspoon to 1 tablespoon): The tip of your thumb is a serving of butter (1 teaspoon), while the length from the knuckle of your thumb to its tip is a serving of salad dressing (1 tablespoon).

Three fingers (4 fluid ounces): Measure three fingers horizontally along the side of a wine glass from the top of the stem. This is approximately one serving of wine.

GET MOVING

Exercise during any weight loss journey is key for revving up your metabolism and boosting your health. However, it doesn't contribute nearly as much to your calories in versus calories out as you might think. Positive nutrition changes are going to be the main driving force for those results.

That said, exercise still plays a critical role in the process. In chapter 2, we'll discuss the benefits of exercise, how it can help with weight loss, and how both cardio and resistance training can be game changers for improving your body composition and enhancing your health. We'll also discuss how overexercising with the intention of getting your calorie burn as high as possible can be counterproductive to weight loss efforts and even damage your health. Finally, while the meal plan in this book aims for 1,200 to 1,500 calories per day, regular exercise will require calorie adjustments, which we'll cover later.

STAY ACCOUNTABLE

Even if you get all of the diet and exercise stuff down, there's one more thing to consider: the mental game that comes with weight loss. Keeping yourself accountable is the key to maintaining all of these new, wonderful health and weight loss habits that you're adopting. There may come a time when you feel like falling off the wagon due to hunger, lack of motivation, or any number of factors. Knowing how to pull yourself out of this slump will give you a smoother road to your goals and long-term success.

One great way to stay accountable is by pursuing this journey with a friend or spouse. Many of the recipes in this book serve multiple people. If you can get the people close to you to adopt the same habits, you're more likely to stick with them. Posting your journey on social media is another good way. Sharing your progress in public allows you to receive encouragement from loved ones and strangers, plus it's a fun, tangible way to track your progress.

QUICK TIPS TO REDUCE CALORIES

There are several easy practices you can adopt to maintain healthy eating and cut down on unnecessary calories:

→ **Avoid empty calories.** It's important to use the calories you *are* eating wisely, so you're sure to get all the nutrition you need despite eating less.

→ **Stay hydrated.** Studies show that people mistake their thirst for hunger about 60 percent of the time. If you aren't drinking enough, you could end up overeating without realizing it. Staying hydrated can help.

→ **Include protein at every meal.** Protein is the macronutrient that keeps you feeling satiated the longest.

→ **Snack on veggies.** Our stomach is a volume counter, not a calorie counter! The stomach can't tell if you just ate 1,000 calories or 400 calories. It only sends a message to the brain when it is full enough. Thus, if you snack on vegetables that are full of water and fiber, you can fill your stomach to satisfaction with fewer calories.

Determining Your Body's Calorie Needs

Individual calorie needs depend on multiple factors. A person's age, weight, height, body composition, activity level, sex, and genetics can all influence their calorie needs. This book's meal plans provide a calorie range to follow for weight loss. Since there is no way for me to provide each reader with a meal plan specific to your own calorie needs, I've provided some tools that can help you estimate your needs and adjust as needed.

One pound of fat equals 3,500 calories. So, if we can create a calorie deficit of 500 calories per day, that equates to a loss of 1 pound per week—a healthy, steady weight loss goal. Here are my estimations of calorie needs per day based on my experience working with weight loss clients:

- Women: 1,200 to 1,500 calories
- Men: 1,700 to 2,000 calories
- Women (exercising 3 times a week or more): 1,400 calories
- Women (exercising 2 times a week or less): 1,200 calories
- Men (exercising 3 times a week or more): 1,800 to 2,000 calories
- Men (exercising 2 times a week or less): 1,700 to 1,900 calories

UNDERSTANDING YOUR BMR

Your BMR (basal metabolic rate) is sometimes referred to as your "metabolism." Your BMR represents how many calories you burn at rest, or how much energy your body uses just to keep you alive. It represents how many calories you burn in order to breathe, keep your heart beating, keep you sitting upright on that couch, send nerve impulses from your brain to your limbs, and digest your food. Your BMR makes up the bulk of your daily calorie burn—activities like exercise are just something a little extra.

You can have your BMR measured by a machine called an indirect calorimeter. However, this method is not easily accessible and can be expensive. In a hospital setting, dietitians will calculate an individual's BMR using the Mifflin-St Jeor equation:

For men: *10 x weight (kg) + 6.25 x height (cm) − 5 x age + 5*

For women: *10 x weight (kg) + 6.25 x height (cm) − 5 x age − 161*

For weight loss to happen, it's necessary to consume fewer calories than your total calorie burn, which includes your BMR plus any additional physical activity.

USING A CALORIE CALCULATOR

A calorie calculator can be a helpful tool—there are many free ones online, and I have one on my Whole Body Reboot website (see Resources, page 161). Though not as accurate as indirect calorimetry, it can be tailored to your goals to give you a ballpark idea of what your needs are.

Your Low-Calorie Kitchen

You probably already have a good idea as to what is "healthy" and what is not. Fast food, fried foods, foods high in added sugar, and overly processed foods aren't necessarily unhealthy, but healthier options are available when trying to lose weight and boost health. These healthier options are prevalent in the recipes in this book. While the following lists are not exhaustive, I've included some healthy food options to stock in your low-calorie kitchen. Separated out by food groups, these foods can be dried, canned, fresh, or frozen, depending on the recipe.

FRUITS AND VEGETABLES

All fruits and vegetables are very healthy for you; however, only 1 out of 10 Americans eats the recommended amount of fruits and vegetables per day. This is a big reason we as a nation struggle with staying healthy and dropping weight. This list is by no means comprehensive but comprises the most common ones included in the recipes of this book. I encourage you to eat a wide variety of fruits and vegetables in order to get all the wonderful phytonutrients and antioxidants they have to offer. Different colors of fruits and vegetables provide different phytonutrients and therefore different health benefits.

FRUITS

- Apples
- Bananas
- Berries (blueberries, strawberries, blackberries, raspberries)
- Citrus (oranges, lemons, limes, grapefruit)
- Kiwi
- Mangos

VEGETABLES

- Asparagus
- Bell pepper
- Broccoli
- Butternut squash
- Carrots
- Cauliflower
- Corn
- Mushrooms
- Onions (red, yellow, white, scallions)
- Potatoes
- Spinach
- Tomatoes
- Zucchini

MEATS AND SEAFOODS

Animal products are great for weight loss, because their protein helps support health and control hunger. Bland, baked chicken breast is far from your only protein choice when eating low calorie! Many lean protein options can be easily incorporated in a weight loss diet. According to the USDA, the classifications of "lean" and "extra lean" are based on the total fat and cholesterol in each serving of beef. Lean beef must have no more than 10 grams of fat, 4.5 grams of saturated fat, and 95 milligrams of cholesterol in a 3.5-ounce serving.

- Beef (sirloin, top round roast, flank steak, etc.)
- Chicken (no skin)
- Eggs
- Pork (lean cuts such as tenderloin, loin, etc.)
- Seafood (shrimp, salmon, mahi-mahi, tilapia, tuna, etc.)
- Turkey

GRAINS, STARCHES, AND LEGUMES

Whole grains are full of vitamins and minerals our bodies need to support health; they also contain fiber to keep us feeling full and keep our digestive tract running smoothly. I've included legumes here, although they fall under the categories of carbohydrate and protein source. Legumes are nutrition powerhouses, making them great for a low-calorie diet.

- Black beans
- Chickpeas (garbanzo beans)
- Farro
- Lentils
- Oats
- Polenta
- Quinoa
- Rice (brown, black, wild)

NUTS, SEEDS, AND GOOD FATS

These foods contain monounsaturated fats, polyunsaturated fats, and some omega-3 fatty acids. These fats are good for your heart and anti-inflammatory, fighting harmful inflammation in your body and helping you burn off that stubborn, visceral belly fat.

- Avocado
- Nuts (almonds, cashews, walnuts, etc.)
- Nut butters (peanut butter, almond butter, etc.)
- Olives
- Oils (avocado, canola, olive)
- Seeds (chia, flaxseed, pumpkin, sunflower, etc.)

DAIRY

Dairy is very good for you. It contains nine essential nutrients as well as high-quality protein. Plant-based beverages like almond milk and oat milk just don't stack up to cow's milk nutritionally, especially in protein. If you have a lactose sensitivity, I recommend lactose-free milk, though not all dairy products contain the same amount of lactose. Milk and ice cream contain the most, while Greek yogurt and hard cheeses like Parmesan contain the least.

- Cottage cheese
- Cow's milk
- Greek yogurt
- Low-fat cheese (less than 6 grams of fat per serving)
- Mozzarella cheese
- Parmesan cheese
- Ricotta cheese

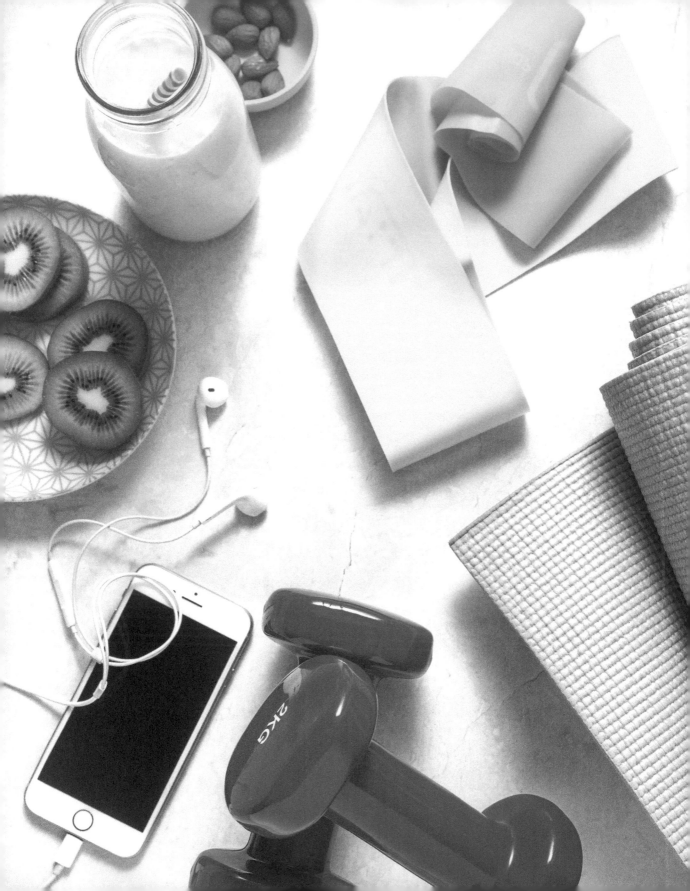

CHAPTER TWO

INCORPORATING EXERCISE

As a responsible health care provider, I understand my limitations. I am not a certified personal trainer, so for this chapter, I consulted my colleague Destini Moody, RD, CSSD. She is a certified personal trainer and board-certified sports dietitian who has worked for MLB, the NBA, and the athletes of the University of California at Berkeley, where she also co-teaches a course about the relationship between exercise and nutrition. This chapter, written by Moody, contains her recommendations. See Resources (page 161) for additional information.

The Health Benefits of Movement

Movement is an underrated health tool in today's often-sedentary society. Like quality nutrition, quality exercise can make a big difference in how your body looks on the outside and how you feel on the inside. Here are five reasons to add movement to your weight loss efforts.

1. **Weight management:** Exercise is not a magic ticket to weight loss—that will come when your nutrition is in order. However, exercise can definitely contribute to your daily calorie burn and prevent further weight gain.

2. **Heart health:** Exercise (especially cardio) is shown to improve cholesterol and decrease the risk of stroke and general heart disease.

3. **Muscle mass and longevity:** After age 30, our muscle mass starts to decline. Science has shown that reduced muscle mass can increase risk of falls, bone breaks, and even early death. Regular weight training can reverse this loss.

4. **Improved energy and mood:** Exercise delivers oxygen to your body's tissues more efficiently, so you'll have more energy to get through the day. Endorphins are also released during exercise, which help you feel happier, less stressed, and more relaxed.

5. **Better sleep:** Regular exercise has been shown to help you sleep better and longer. Just don't exercise right before bed, or your endorphins will keep you too hyped up to get to sleep.

Exercising and Low-Calorie Living

It's no surprise—exercise is good for your health and can help with your weight loss goals. However, when eating low calorie, you must be careful. Eating low calorie creates a calorie deficit. Exercise contributes to that deficit, and if you do too much exercise while eating too few calories, you will begin doing more harm to your body than good.

I have seen far too many clients who were overexercising, thinking they were doing the right thing, but they were actually harming their body and their progress. Too much exercise can cause muscle loss, muscle weakness, reduced appetite, inability to get through a workout, loss of sleep, and even depression. Weight loss is great, but it means nothing if you're sacrificing your health for it.

The other part of the equation is to ensure your workouts are consistent. If you only put forth half the effort, you'll only get half the benefits. So, not too much, not too little. Feeling like Goldilocks yet? Not to worry—here are some best practices you can follow to make sure you're in the exercising sweet spot.

CREATE A REGULAR ROUTINE

As a personal trainer, the person I see canceling their gym membership just two months in is the person who goes in five days a week, but without a plan. They wander from machine to dumbbell to barbell, doing half-hearted lifts for random muscle groups, but with no real rhyme, reason, or structure to their daily routine. They have no scheduled "off" days and instead go whenever they feel like it (and stay home when they don't).

Not having a plan will sabotage the ability to construct a habit around exercise. Just exercising when you feel like it is not a sustainable approach. A plan keeps you accountable and provides a clear structure to follow, with goals to meet. Use a note-taking app on your phone or use pen and paper to record your exercises. Record how much weight you lifted or how many jumps you did, and see how much stronger you get and how your endurance improves from week to week. Also, decide ahead of time which days of the week you plan to exercise and schedule it in your calendar like you would any other obligation. This will do wonders for your morale and give you the drive to keep going.

Investing in a gym membership can be life-changing, but there's also no shortage of fitness apps and YouTube channels, so just find one you can stick with! Even if you're not deadlifting 500 pounds, moving your body in some form daily (even just walking or some light morning jogging) will benefit you.

BALANCE CARDIO AND STRENGTH

Despite the widespread myth, tons of cardio is not the essential element of losing weight. Most bodybuilders will tell you to avoid cardio if you don't want to lose your hard-earned muscle gains and strength. The truth? It's somewhere in the middle. Yes, cardio can promote fat loss, but only if done right. However, cardio will contribute little to helping you get stronger, and too much can indeed make you weaker and break down your muscle tissue. This is why it's optimal to include a balance of cardio and strength exercises to reap the benefits of both without suffering the consequences of excess.

Cardio: High-intensity interval training (HIIT) is the most effective type of cardio for losing fat and usually requires no equipment. Examples of HIITs include burpees, jump rope, stair drills, power jumps, and even jumping jacks. This approach helps burn fat while also preserving muscle. Running on the treadmill or the elliptical for an hour straight is going to give you a decent calorie burn, but that type of "steady-state" cardio also uses up your muscle tissue for energy. Another thing that makes HIIT different is that, instead of one long, sustained bout of exercise, you have short bursts of very intense exercise with short rests in between. This pattern of exercise is proven to burn calories faster than cardio that is steady-state. Therefore, 20 to 30 minutes of HIIT a minimum of 2 times a week is a good recommendation for losing fat. There is no need to track your heart rate, as there is no solid evidence that a certain heart rate puts you in a "fat-burning" zone.

Strength/Resistance Training: Strength training is not just for getting bigger muscles. It may not pack the heart-healthy punch that cardio does, but it does give you the benefits we talked about earlier (see The Health Benefits of Movement, page 16) and makes you stronger. You also burn more calories after exercise from lifting weights; that is, your body keeps burning after the lifting is done. This is called EPOC, or excess postexercise oxygen consumption. Strength training is recommended no more than 1 hour a day for a minimum of 3 days a week.

FITNESS MYTHS

Before we get into the workout plan, let's debunk some of the most common fitness myths that hold folks back from results.

Myth 1: You can spot-reduce. Any fitness guru who has tried to tell you there are certain exercises you can do to get rid of your love handles or trim your inner thighs was probably trying to sell you something expensive! The fact is, the body can't select where it burns fat. If you want to slim a certain place, you need to lose fat all over first.

Myth 2: It's best to work out on an empty stomach. It's very important to keep your body fueled despite eating low calorie. Yes, keeping a calorie deficit is important for weight loss, but if you haven't eaten enough beforehand to put in a solid enough workout for a decent calorie burn, you're wasting your time in the gym.

Myth 3: Women should lift lighter weights than men. Some women are scared away from strength training because they think they'll get "bulky." Take it from me, someone who has been actively *trying* to bulk up her upper body for years: Most women just don't have the testosterone men have to get bulky and will still want to lift heavy to boost calorie burn!

Myth 4: You need to work out to "earn" your food. The ability to enjoy both your food and your exercise are key to truly living a healthy life, so please reject this toxic ideology. It's just not a practical way to approach exercise and weight loss.

MAKE TIME FOR REST AND RECOVERY

What's more important than exercise itself? Recovery!

The "no days off" mentality is well-intentioned but also harmful. You see, exercise puts the body through a lot of stress—in fact, we damage our muscles in order to make them grow. However, they only grow if we allow them to recover from this damage. If we don't let them recover, they stay broken down, we lose muscle, and we lose strength. Thus, much of our exercise is wasted.

Resting is also important for mental health. It will do wonders for you to just take a day off from the obligation of the gym, so you can use that time to do activities you love with friends or family, or just for some good old "me" time. If you reward yourself with rest, you're less likely to burn out, and exercise will be more of a joy than a dreaded everyday commitment. At least 1 or 2 days off a week from exercise is highly recommended.

FUEL YOUR BODY WELL

There's more to recovery than taking days off. Refueling your body properly after exercise is key, too. Many people on a low-calorie diet end up eating too little for their body to run efficiently, especially when they're increasing their calorie burn from exercise.

Calories aren't just a unit of measurement we use to see how much weight we are gaining or losing. Food is the very essence of our energy, strength, and function. We need calories to exercise, as well as to accomplish everyday activities like playing with our kids, working, and even playing video games. Other latent bodily processes also require calories to keep our heart beating, our lungs inhaling and exhaling, and our brain functioning.

The Exercises

The exercises recommended here are only a few examples of exercises you can incorporate into your weight loss routine. Even though getting into the gym for an exercise program gives you access to a wide range of equipment, which will yield a higher calorie burn, this chapter includes exercises that you can also do at home if you don't have access to a gym or equipment. If you have access to equipment, perform the following exercises with weights when indicated.

If you have heart disease or other heart issues, diabetes, kidney disease, asthma or another respiratory ailment, or osteoporosis, please talk to your doctor before beginning any exercise program.

LOWER BODY EXERCISES

Squats

Target the quads (front of the legs) and glutes (butt).

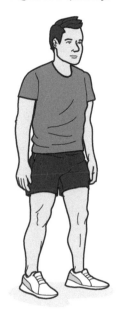

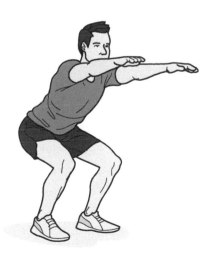

1. Stand with your feet hip-width apart, toes pointed forward.

2. Bend your knees and hinge at your hips to sit your butt back and down as if you're sitting into a chair. Keep your chest lifted and spine long; do not arch your back. Do not let your knees come past your toes or fall inward toward one another. You can lift your arms in front of your chest for stability.

3. Stop when your thighs are parallel to the ground and your knees are at a 90-degree angle. (If you can go deeper without bending your spine or compromising your form, do so.)

4. Press the floor away through your heels to drive yourself back up into a standing position. Repeat.

Recommended reps: Do 12 squats in a set and perform 3 sets.

Add weight: Add weight by holding a barbell on the shoulders, two dumbbells at your sides, or a single dumbbell in front of your chest with both hands.

Lunges

Target the quads (front of the legs), hamstrings (back of the legs), and glutes (butt).

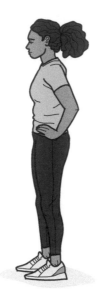

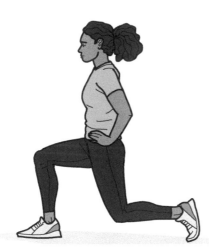

1. Stand with your feet hip-width apart, toes pointed forward. Place your hands on your hips for balance.

2. Step forward with your right leg like you are taking a large step. The heel of your back (left) foot should be off the ground.

3. Bend both your knees to 90 degrees and lunge straight down. Do not push your front knee over your toes or lunge forward. Keep your front (right) knee over your front (right) ankle and your chest lifted and spine straight. Your shoulders should be in line with your hips.

4. Press into your front (right) heel to rise up and step back into your starting stance. Repeat with your opposite leg.

Recommended reps: Do 10 lunges on each leg for a total of 20 lunges per set. Perform 3 sets.

Add weight: When you get used to doing the movement properly, add weight by holding a barbell on the shoulders, two dumbbells at your sides, or a single dumbbell in front of your chest with both hands.

Burpees

Target the quads (front of the legs), glutes (butt), and shoulders.

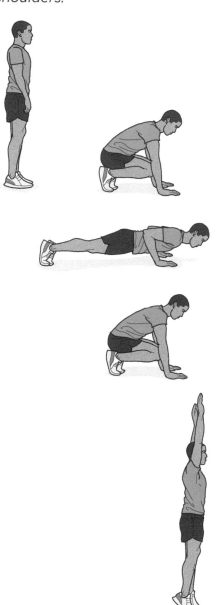

1. Stand with your feet shoulder-width apart, weight in your heels.

2. Sit your hips back and bend your knees to come to a low squat. Place your hands on the floor in front of your feet.

3. Shift your weight onto your hands and jump your feet back to land softly on the balls of your feet in a high-plank position. Engage your core; do not let your back sag or your hips pike up.

4. Jump your feet forward so they land outside your hands in that low squat position.

5. Drive through your heels to explosively stand up and jump into the air as you reach your arms overhead.

6. Land softly, bending your knees to absorb the impact, and repeat immediately.

Recommended reps: Do 10 burpees as a set and perform 3 sets with 1 minute of rest in between sets.

UPPER-BODY EXERCISES

Push-Ups

Target the chest and front of the shoulders.

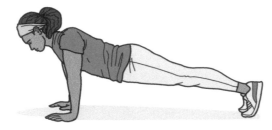

1. Start with your hands on the floor slightly wider than shoulder-width apart and in line with your chest, arms fully extended. Your toes should be on the ground, feet hip-width apart.

2. Keep your neck neutral and gaze slightly forward at the ground in front of you. Do not tuck your chin or look up straight ahead. Your body should create one long line from head to heels.

3. Actively press your palms into the floor and engage your thighs and core as if holding a plank to keep the lower body stiff throughout the exercises.

4. Bend your elbows back at 45-degree angles to lower your body toward the floor. Do not let your elbows flare out to the sides. (You should look like an arrow, not a T.)

5. Pause when your chest is barely touching the floor.

6. Exhale and press into your hands to push your body away from the floor as one unit (hips and shoulders in one line) to return to the starting position. Repeat.

Recommended reps: Do 10 to 20 push-ups as a set and perform 3 sets.

Triceps Dips

Target the triceps (back of the upper arms).

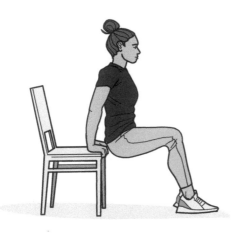

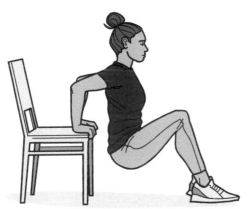

1. Sit with your palms on the floor behind you and at your sides and your knees bent at 90 degrees, feet flat on the floor.

2. Angle your palms so your fingertips are pointing forward. Raise your hips off the ground into the starting position. (You will only be using your arms for resistance; do not use your hips or legs during this exercise.)

3. Bend your elbows back (not out to the side), and lower your body toward the ground until you feel tension in the back of your upper arms.

4. Straighten your arms to the starting position and repeat. To increase difficulty, straighten your legs so only the bottoms of your heels are on the ground. You can also use a chair, bench, or other flat elevated surface to place your palms on, and perform these dips by lowering your butt toward the floor as you bend your elbows. Do not let your shoulders cave inward; keep your chest lifted and core engaged.

Recommended reps: Do 15 to 20 triceps dips as a set and perform 3 sets.

Biceps Curls

Target the biceps (front of the upper arms).

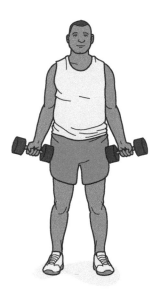

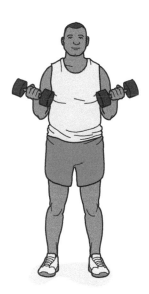

1. Stand with your feet shoulder-width apart, arms at your sides and palms facing forward.

2. Tightly grip a dumbbell, a barbell, or something heavy (like a water jug or a bottle of laundry detergent) in either hand.

3. Keeping your core tight, bend your elbows and bring your wrists toward your upper chest and stop when you feel maximum tension in the front of your arms, stopping the weights just in front of your shoulders. Keep your elbows next to your waist throughout the movement; do not let them swing forward.

4. Squeeze the biceps at the top and hold for 3 seconds, then slowly reverse the movement to bring both arms back down to your sides. Repeat.

Recommended reps: Do 12 biceps curls as a set and perform 3 sets.

CORE EXERCISES

High Plank

Targets all the core (trunk) muscles.

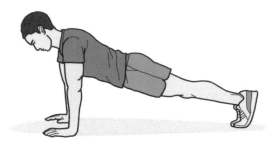

1. Start with your hands on the floor under your shoulders, arms fully extended like you're about to do a push-up, and your toes on the floor, feet hip-width apart.

2. Squeeze your glutes to stabilize your body and neutralize your neck and spine. Your head should be in line with your back, creating one long line from head to heels. Keep your body straight, like a plank. Don't let your butt stick up too far in the air or let your hips sink too close to the ground.

3. Hold for 20 seconds, remembering to breathe and tighten your core.

Recommended reps: Hold for 20 seconds, rest, and repeat 3 to 5 times.

Flutter Kicks

Target the lower abdominals.

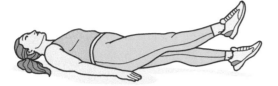

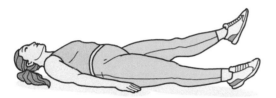

1. Lie on your back and extend your legs up off the floor at a 45-degree angle.

2. Keep your arms on the floor at your sides, palms down. Lift your head, neck, and shoulders slightly off the ground, but do not tuck your chin.

3. Keep your legs straight and your toes pointed. Lower one leg, then raise that leg as you lower the other. Continue alternating lowering and lifting your legs to "flutter" your legs.

Recommended reps: Flutter for 30 seconds as a set and perform 4 sets.

Mountain Climbers

Target the upper and lower abdominals.

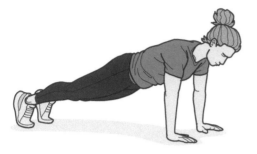

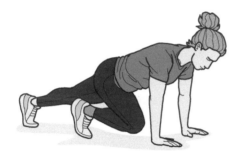

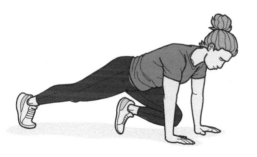

1. Start with your hands on the floor under your shoulders, arms fully extended like you're about to do a push-up, and your toes on the floor, feet hip-width apart. Keep your spine long and engage your core.

2. Pull your right knee in toward your right elbow.

3. Send the right foot back to the starting position as you simultaneously pull your left knee in toward your left elbow. Return your left foot to the starting position.

4. Continue alternating driving each knee in toward your chest and begin to pick up the pace until it feels like you're running in place in that high-plank position.

Recommended reps: Perform for 30 seconds for a set, rest for 1 minute, and repeat for a total of 4 sets.

Sample Workout Plan

Here is a sample workout plan that you can use to kick-start your workout routine. It is recommended that you take two days off from intense workouts, but if you'd like some sort of movement, light yoga, walks, or just stretching are acceptable on your rest days.

This combined strength training and cardio plan, in conjunction with your low-calorie eating, will position you for success in your weight loss ventures as long as you stay consistent. If you are more of an advanced weight lifter, check out more detailed workout plans at TheAthletesDietitian.com.

Monday: Strength training: Upper body

Tuesday: Cardio *(HIIT, cycling, running, swimming)*

Wednesday: Rest day

Thursday: Strength training: Lower body

Friday: Cardio *(HIIT, cycling, running, swimming)*

Saturday: Strength training: Core

Sunday: Rest day

To get the best muscle adaptation and maximum calorie burn on your strength days, rest no longer than 45 to 60 seconds between sets. With cardio, it is recommended to go through your movement either at 30 seconds on with 1 minute of rest, or 1 minute on with 2 minutes of rest, depending on the difficulty of the movement.

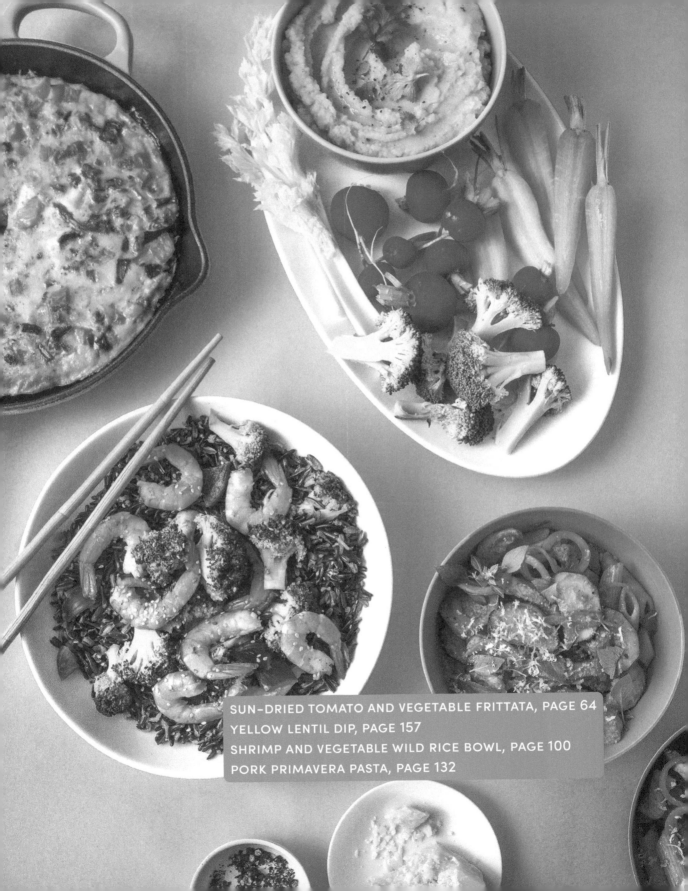

SUN-DRIED TOMATO AND VEGETABLE FRITTATA, PAGE 64
YELLOW LENTIL DIP, PAGE 157
SHRIMP AND VEGETABLE WILD RICE BOWL, PAGE 100
PORK PRIMAVERA PASTA, PAGE 132

CHAPTER THREE

THE MEAL PLAN

The meal plans in this chapter are your blueprint for low-calorie eating. Here, we've taken the delicious recipes in coming chapters and created a daily menu for you to follow, making staying within your calorie goals practically foolproof. Here's what you can expect from this meal plan:

- The meal plan will guide you over 28 days.
- The meal plan serves one person and makes smart use of leftovers so you don't waste any food.
- You won't find yourself cooking every single day. My goal when making these meal plans was for you to cook once and eat multiple times; having meals already prepared can be key to sticking to your plan and avoiding impulse eating.
- All the ingredients are familiar and easy to find and are reused across recipes to avoid food waste or overspending at the grocery store.
- Every meal plan includes a total daily calories column (an average of 1,350) depending on your individual needs. If you are a woman who exercises more than three days a week, you should increase your daily calories to 1,400 for fuel. Additionally, for men, your calories should be closer to 1,800 per day.
- If you need to bump up your calories, double a side, add an extra snack, or add dessert. If you need to bulk up your meals, simply double the portion of one of your meals, double one of the snacks, or add a second snack to your day. Everything is labeled for you, so a quick calculation will determine how to reach your calorie goal.
- Conversely, if you need to lower your calorie intake, you can remove the snacks or dessert.

Week 1

Many people get discouraged after their first shopping trip when starting a new meal plan. This is because, in week 1, your shopping list will be the longest and probably most expensive with all of the spices and other staples you'll be stocking up on to prepare for the weeks to come. Keep in mind that many of these items will not be needed in the subsequent weeks because they'll last you a while. Toward the end of week 4, revisit your shopping list for longer-lasting ingredients like oils and spices to see if you need to replenish your supply.

To prep for success for this week, you can prepare a batch of the Basic Brown Rice (page 150).

Week 1 Meal Plan

	BREAKFAST	LUNCH	DINNER	SNACK	TOTAL CALORIES
Monday	Sun-Dried Tomato and Vegetable Frittata (page 64)............ 303 1 cup blueberries 85	Salmon Cakes Salad (page 90)..........271 ½ cup Basic Brown Rice (page 150)........129	Ground Turkey and Vegetable Stuffed Bell Peppers (page 118)........ 302 *Leftover* ½ cup Basic Brown Rice 129	Applesauce with Seeds (page 138) 123	1,342
Tuesday	Creamy Green Smoothie (page 57)............ 315	Roast Beef and Cheese Panini (page 79)..........299	Sheet Pan Mediterranean Chicken with Butternut Squash (page 109)......... 225 1 ounce dark chocolate (at least 75% dark) 160	Mini Parfait (page 137) 204	1,203
Wednesday	*Leftover* Sun-Dried Tomato and Vegetable Frittata .... 303 1 cup blueberries 85	*Leftover* Salmon Cakes Salad ....271 *Leftover* ½ cup Basic Brown Rice 129	*Leftover* Ground Turkey and Vegetable Stuffed Bell Peppers .... 302 *Leftover* ½ cup Basic Brown Rice 129	Applesauce with Seeds (page 138) 123	1,342

	BREAKFAST	LUNCH	DINNER	SNACK	TOTAL CALORIES
Thursday	Creamy Green Smoothie (page 57) 315	*Leftover* Roast Beef and Cheese Panini 299	*Leftover* Ground Turkey and Vegetable Stuffed Bell Peppers .... 302 *Leftover* ½ cup Basic Brown Rice 129 1 ounce dark chocolate (at least 75% dark) 160	¾ cup blueberries + 12 almonds 150	1,355
Friday	Superfood Parfait (page 58) 368	*Leftover* Salmon Cakes Salad ....271 *Leftover* ½ cup Basic Brown Rice 129	*Leftover* Sheet Pan Mediterranean Chicken with Butternut Squash .... 225 1 ounce dark chocolate (at least 75% dark) 160	Applesauce with Seeds (page 138) 123	1,276
Saturday	*Leftover* Sun-Dried Tomato and Vegetable Frittata .... 303 1 cup blueberries 85	Avocado, Tomato, and Poached Egg Toast (page 78) 229	*Leftover* Ground Turkey and Vegetable Stuffed Bell Peppers .... 302 ½ cup Basic Brown Rice (page 150) 129	Ricotta à la Méditerranée (page 143) 229	1,277
Sunday	*Leftover* Sun-Dried Tomato and Vegetable Frittata .... 303 1 cup blueberries 85	*Leftover* Salmon Cakes Salad ....271 *Leftover* ½ cup Basic Brown Rice 129	*Leftover* Sheet Pan Mediterranean Chicken with Butternut Squash .... 225 1-ounce dark chocolate (at least 75% dark) 160	¾ cup blueberries + 12 almonds 150	1,323

Shopping List

PRODUCE

FRESH

- Arugula, 1 (5-ounce) bag
- Avocado, medium (1)
- Bell pepper, orange (1)
- Bell peppers, any color (4)
- Bell peppers, red (2)
- Blueberries (6 cups)
- Butternut squash, cubed (1 pound)
- Celery stalks (2)
- Cherry tomatoes (2 cups)
- Cucumber (1)
- Lemons (2)
- Onions, red (2)
- Onion, yellow (1)
- Orange (1)
- Parsley (1 bunch)
- Pineapple, sliced (1 cup)
- Scallions (11)
- Spinach, 1 (5-ounce) bag
- Tomatoes, medium (2)
- Zucchini (1)

FROZEN

- Mixed berries (5 cups)
- Mixed vegetables (carrots, corn, and green beans) (2 cups)
- Peas (1 cup)

EGGS AND DAIRY

- Eggs, large (12)
- Greek yogurt, plain, 2% (2 cups)
- Jarlsberg cheese slices, lite (2 ounces)
- Ricotta cheese, part-skim (8 ounces)

MEAT, POULTRY, AND SEAFOOD

- Chicken breasts, boneless, skinless (1 pound)
- Ground turkey, lean (1 pound)
- Roast beef, deli-sliced (4 ounces)

PANTRY

DRIED HERBS AND SPICES

- Black pepper, freshly ground
- Cinnamon, ground
- Cinnamon sticks
- Cloves, ground
- Garlic powder
- Oregano, dried
- Sea salt
- Thyme, dried

JARRED, BOTTLED, BAGGED, AND CANNED

- Almonds, raw, 1 (16-ounce) bag
- Applesauce, unsweetened, 1 (24-ounce) jar
- Bread, light, whole-grain (~70 calories per slice), 1 loaf
- Broth, chicken or vegetable, 1 (32-ounce) carton
- Canola oil
- Cacao nibs, 1 (8-ounce) bag
- Chia seeds, 1 (8-ounce) bag
- Dark chocolate, 75% or more (4 ounces)
- Figs, dried, 1 (7-ounce) bag
- Flaxseed, 1 (16-ounce) bag
- Garlic, crushed, 1 (9-ounce) bottle
- Ginger, crushed, 1 (4¼-ounce) bottle
- Honey
- Monk fruit sweetener, 1 (8.29 ounce) bag
- Mustard
- Nonstick cooking spray
- Pumpkin seeds, raw, 1 (8-ounce) bag
- Oats, dry, 1-minute, 1 (18-ounce) bag or container
- Olive oil, extra-virgin
- Protein powder (whey, soy, or pea)*, 1 (5-pound) container
- Rice, brown, dry, 1 (14-ounce) bag
- Salmon, Alaskan pink, skinless, boneless, no salt added, 3 (6-ounce) cans
- Sesame seeds, 1 (3¾-ounce) jar
- Sun-dried tomatoes, not in oil (1 package)
- Tomatoes, diced, 1 (14½-ounce) can
- Walnuts, crushed, 1 (8-ounce) bag
- Whole-kernel corn, 1 (15¼-ounce) can

*When choosing a protein powder (whey, soy, pea, or rice), look for one with at least 20 grams of protein and 2 grams or less of sugar per scoop.

Week 2

This week we'll be changing it up with your meals and snacks, so you won't get "food fatigue" from eating the same things week in and week out. My hope is that you are getting settled into the habit of adhering to a meal plan. Please note that, just like in the previous week, the calories are not exactly the same every day. This is okay—it's not the day-to-day calories that matter but the weekly average. Even if you overeat one day, this will make no impact on your weight as long as your weekly average of calories still allows you to stay in your calorie deficit. That's why these meal plans work on a weekly average to give you more flexibility with your meals while still keeping you on track.

This week, get ahead by preparing the Basic Flavorful Quinoa (page 151), the Lemon-Mustard Vinaigrette (page 155), and a double batch of Chia Cacao Pudding (page 142).

Week 2 Meal Plan

	BREAKFAST	LUNCH	DINNER	SNACK	TOTAL CALORIES
Monday	Crustless Egg and Spinach Quiches (page 66) 335	Chicken Cilantro Patties (page 89) .... 151 3 cups mixed greens + ½ cup cherry tomatoes + ½ cup can chickpeas .... 94 Lemon-Mustard Vinaigrette (page 155) 45	Sheet Pan Glazed Balsamic Salmon with Asparagus (page 105) .... 230 ½ cup Basic Flavorful Quinoa (page 151) .... 123 Chia Cacao Pudding (page 142) 144	Mixed Dried Fruit with Parmesan Cheese (page 136) 215	1,337
Tuesday	Warm Apple-Spiced Smoothie (page 54) 299	Turkey Spinach Roll (page 80) .... 398 1 orange 60	*Leftover* Sheet Pan Glazed Balsamic Salmon with Asparagus .... 230 *Leftover* ½ cup Basic Flavorful Quinoa 123	Yellow Lentil Dip with Olives and Red Peppers (page 141) 257	1,367

	BREAKFAST	LUNCH	DINNER	SNACK	TOTAL CALORIES
Wednesday	*Leftover* Crustless Egg and Spinach Quiches....335	*Leftover* Chicken Cilantro Patties ... 151 3 cups mixed greens + ½ cup cherry tomatoes + ½ cup can chickpeas .... 94 *Leftover* Lemon-Mustard Vinaigrette........................... 45	Vegetable-Layered Cheese Lasagna (page 127)........... 394 *Leftover* Chia Cacao Pudding 144	Mixed Dried Fruit with Parmesan Cheese (page 136) 215	1,378
Thursday	Warm Apple-Spiced Smoothie (page 54) 299	Turkey Spinach Roll (page 80)............................. 398 1 orange............................. 60	*Leftover* Sheet Pan Glazed Balsamic Salmon with Asparagus ... 230 *Leftover* ½ cup Basic Flavorful Quinoa 123	Mixed Dried Fruit with Parmesan Cheese (page 136) 215	1,325
Friday	*Leftover* Crustless Egg and Spinach Quiches....335	*Leftover* Chicken Cilantro Patties ... 151 3 cups mixed greens + ½ cup cherry tomatoes + ½ cup can chickpeas .... 94 *Leftover* Lemon-Mustard Vinaigrette 45	*Leftover* Vegetable-Layered Cheese Lasagna .... 394 Chia Cacao Pudding (page 142).......................... 144	*Leftover* Yellow Lentil Dip with Olives and Red Peppers 257	1,420
Saturday	*Leftover* Crustless Egg and Spinach Quiches....335	Turkey Spinach Roll (page 80)............................. 398 1 orange............................. 60	*Leftover* Sheet Pan Glazed Balsamic Salmon with Asparagus ... 230 *Leftover* ½ cup Basic Flavorful Quinoa 123	*Leftover* Yellow Lentil Dip with Olives and Red Peppers 257	1,403
Sunday	¾ cup 2% Greek yogurt + 8 strawberries + 1 tablespoon chopped walnuts + 1 teaspoon honey 255	*Leftover* Chicken Cilantro Patties ... 151 3 cups mixed greens + ½ cup cherry tomatoes + ½ cup can chickpeas .... 94 *Leftover* Lemon-Mustard Vinaigrette........................... 45	*Leftover* Vegetable-Layered Cheese Lasagna .... 394 *Leftover* Chia Cacao Pudding 144	*Leftover* Yellow Lentil Dip with Olives and Red Peppers 257	1,340

Shopping List

PRODUCE

FRESH

- Asparagus (16 spears)
- Basil (1 bunch)
- Bell pepper, red (2)
- Carrots, shredded (½ cup)
- Cherry tomatoes (2 cups)
- Cilantro (1 bunch)
- Eggplant (1)
- Lemons (4)
- Mixed leafy greens (12 cups)
- Mushrooms, baby bella (2 cups)
- Onion, yellow (1)
- Oranges (3)
- Scallions (5)
- Spinach, 1 (5-ounce) bag
- Strawberries (1 pound)
- Zucchini (3)

FROZEN

- Spinach (3 cups)

EGGS AND DAIRY

- Eggs, large (12)
- Greek yogurt, plain, 2% (1 cup)
- Milk, 1% (2 cups)
- Feta cheese (3 ounces)
- Jarlsberg cheese slices, lite (3 ounces)
- Mozzarella cheese, part-skim, shredded (1 cup)
- Parmesan cheese (1½ cups)
- Parmesan cheese, block (3 ounces)
- Ricotta cheese, part-skim (3 cups)

MEAT, POULTRY, AND SEAFOOD

- Chicken breasts, boneless, skinless (1 pound)
- Ground chicken, lean (1 pound)
- Turkey, deli-sliced (4 ounces)
- Salmon, boneless and skinless fillets (1 pound)

PANTRY

DRIED HERBS AND SPICES

- Basil, dry
- Cinnamon, ground
- Cumin, ground
- Umami seasoning

JARRED, BOTTLED, BAGGED, AND CANNED

- Apricots, dried, 1 (7-ounce) bag
- Balsamic vinegar, glaze, 1 (8½-ounce) bottle
- Broth, chicken or vegetable, 1 (32-ounce) carton
- Cacao powder, 1 (8-ounce) bag
- Chickpeas, 2 (15½-ounce) cans
- Cornstarch, 1 box
- Honey
- Lavash bread, whole-grain, 3 (10- by 8-inch) rounds
- Lentils, yellow, dry, 1 (16-ounce) bag
- Mayonnaise, avocado-oil based, 1 (24-ounce) jar
- Olives, kalamata, 1 (5-ounce) bottle or can
- Prunes, dried, 1 (7-ounce) bag
- Quinoa, dry, 1 (8-ounce) bag
- Rice crackers, 1 (8-ounce) bag or container
- Stevia In The Raw, granulated, 1 (9.7-ounce) bag
- Tomatoes, diced, 1 (14½-ounce) can
- Tomato paste, 1 (6-ounce) can

Week 3

In week 3, we get into some low-calorie comfort food dishes like savory ham and egg breakfast muffins, fried rice, and even pizza! Even though these meals have a reputation for being calorie-dense, cooking your meals at home lets you control both the flavor and calorie content. This way, you can enjoy your favorite dishes healthfully. If I choose a recipe to put in the plan, I try my best to use it throughout the week. Remember, if you have leftover servings after the plan is done, you can always freeze them. For example, the Fried Shrimp Brown Rice (page 110) freezes very well and can be reheated as a backup dinner in a pinch!

To get ahead this week, prepare the Steamed Broccoli and Cauliflower with Lemon Juice (page 152) and the High-Protein Overnight Oats (page 60). You'll have some leftovers beyond the plan. Share the Overnight Oats with a friend or family member or freeze it; use the leftovers for "bulk it up" snacks as calories allow. You can also freeze fresh vegetables, like arugula, for future use!

Week 3 Meal Plan

	BREAKFAST	LUNCH	DINNER	SNACKS	TOTAL CALORIES
Monday	Egg, Cheese, and Ham English Muffins (page 68) 298	Turkey Meatball Quinoa Soup (page 94) .... 315 1 large orange 85	Fried Shrimp Brown Rice (page 110) .... 342 Steamed Broccoli and Cauliflower with Lemon Juice (page 152) 72	3 cups air-popped popcorn seasoned with 1 teaspoon olive oil and sprinkle of sea salt + 1 light string cheese 190	1,302
Tuesday	*Leftover* Egg, Cheese, and Ham English Muffins 298	*Leftover* Turkey Meatball Quinoa Soup 315 1 large orange 85	*Leftover* Fried Shrimp Brown Rice .... 342 *Leftover* Steamed Broccoli and Cauliflower with Lemon Juice 72	1 medium apple + 18 almonds 220	1,332

	BREAKFAST	LUNCH	DINNER	SNACKS	TOTAL CALORIES
Wednesday	High-Protein Overnight Oats (page 60) 246	Curried Chicken Pita Wrap (page 81) .... 454 12 medium strawberries.... 60	*Leftover* Turkey Meatball Quinoa Soup .... 315 1 ounce dark chocolate (at least 75% dark).... 160	3 cups air-popped popcorn seasoned with 1 teaspoon olive oil and sprinkle of sea salt + 1 light string cheese 190	1,425
Thursday	*Leftover* High-Protein Overnight Oats 246	*Leftover* Curried Chicken Pita Wrap ...... 454 1 large orange 85	*Leftover* Fried Shrimp Brown Rice .... 342 *Leftover* Steamed Broccoli and Cauliflower with Lemon Juice 72	1 medium apple + 18 almonds.......... 220	1,419
Friday	*Leftover* Egg, Cheese, and Ham English Muffins.......... 298	*Leftover* Turkey Meatball Quinoa Soup 315 12 medium strawberries.... 60	*Leftover* Fried Shrimp Brown Rice .... 342 *Leftover* Steamed Broccoli and Cauliflower with Lemon Juice 72	3 cups air-popped popcorn seasoned with 1 teaspoon olive oil and sprinkle of sea salt + 1 light string cheese 190	1,277
Saturday	*Leftover* Egg, Cheese, and Ham English Muffins.......... 298	*Leftover* Curried Chicken Pita Wrap ...... 454 12 medium strawberries.... 60	Sheet Pan Cracked-Egg Pizza (page 108) 480	1 medium apple + 18 almonds.......... 220	1,512
Sunday	*Leftover* High-Protein Overnight Oats............... 246	*Leftover* Curried Chicken Pita Wrap ...... 454 1 large orange 85	*Leftover* Sheet Pan Cracked-Egg Pizza 480	1 medium apple + 18 almonds.......... 220	1,485

Shopping List

PRODUCE

FRESH

- Apples, medium (4)
- Arugula, 1 (5-ounce) bag
- Bell pepper, red (1)
- Bell pepper, yellow (1)
- Broccoli (1 head)
- Carrots (2)
- Cauliflower (1 head)
- Celery (6 stalks)
- Cilantro (1 bunch)
- Lemons (2)
- Oranges, large (4)
- Onion, red (1)
- Scallions (9)
- Strawberries, 3 pounds
- Zucchini (1)

FROZEN

- Berries (2 cups)
- Peas (1 cup)

EGGS AND DAIRY

- Eggs, large (12)
- Greek yogurt, plain, 2% (2½ cups)
- Jarlsberg cheese slices, lite (4 ounces)
- Milk, 1% (2 cups)
- Mozzarella cheese, part-skim, shredded (3 ounces)
- String cheese, light (6)

MEAT, POULTRY, AND SEAFOOD

- Canadian bacon (2 ounces)
- Chicken breasts, boneless, skinless (1 pound)
- Ground turkey, lean (1 pound)
- Shrimp, peeled and deveined (1 pound)

PANTRY

DRIED HERBS AND SPICES

- Curry powder

JARRED, BOTTLED, BAGGED, AND CANNED

- Broth, chicken or vegetable, 1 (32-ounce) carton
- Cashews, salted (¼ cup)
- Dark chocolate, 75% (1 ounce)
- English muffins, whole-grain (4)
- Pitas, whole-grain, 4 (6½-inch)
- Pizza sauce, 1 (6-ounce) can
- Popcorn kernels, 1 (30-ounce) jar
- Raisins (¼ cup)
- Sesame oil
- Soy sauce, reduced-sodium
- Tomatoes, diced, 1 (14½-ounce) can

Week 4

This final week of your meal plan is close to my heart, as it includes many dishes from my home country of Peru and mixes up your meals with a fun variety of cuisines. At this point, you should be pretty awesome at meal planning, so take the time to applaud yourself! Making meal prep a habit can be the hardest part of a low-calorie lifestyle for most people, but as you've likely noticed, it is a game changer in terms of making healthy eating happen. If you've been sticking to the meal plans and exercise programming, you're probably feeling more energized and perhaps even seeing results. If you've liked the way you've been eating and feeling these last few weeks, feel free to start again and try all of the delicious recipes in this book.

Get ahead this week by preparing the Roasted Vegetables (page 154) and the Basic Brown Rice (page 150).

Week 4 Meal Plan

	BREAKFAST	LUNCH	DINNER	SNACKS	TOTAL CALORIES
Monday	Egg and Avocado Burrito (page 70).......280 1 cup diced cantaloupe......60	Black Bean, Corn, and Chicken Sausage Bowl (page 98)............338 1 medium apple....................95	Ground Turkey and Vegetable Stuffed Bell Peppers (page 118)................................302 1½ cups Roasted Vegetables (page 154)................................79 ½ cup Basic Brown Rice (page 150)...............................129	Mini Parfait (page 137) 204	1,487
Tuesday	*Leftover* Egg and Avocado Burrito...........280 1 cup diced cantaloupe......60	Fish Tacos with Mango and Kiwi Salsa (page 84)............438	*Leftover* Ground Turkey and Vegetable Stuffed Bell Peppers..............302 *Leftover* 1½ cups Roasted Vegetables................................79 *Leftover* ½ cup Basic Brown Rice 129	25 grapes + 2 light string cheeses......190	1,478

	BREAKFAST	LUNCH	DINNER	SNACKS	TOTAL CALORIES
Wednesday	Berry Mango Bliss Smoothie (page 56).......332	*Leftover* Fish Tacos with Mango and Kiwi Salsa 438	Seafood à la Paella with Farro (page 111)...............................281 1 ounce dark chocolate (at least 75% dark)...............160	Mason Jar Roasted Vegetable Soup with Parmesan Cheese (page 140) 115	1,326
Thursday	*Leftover* Egg and Avocado Burrito...........280 1 cup diced cantaloupe......60	*Leftover* Black Bean, Corn, and Chicken Sausage Bowl....338 1 medium apple ..95	*Leftover* Seafood à la Paella with Farro ....281 1 ounce dark chocolate (at least 75% dark).................160	25 grapes + 2 light string cheeses 190	1,404
Friday	Berry Mango Bliss Smoothie (page 56).......332	*Leftover* Fish Tacos with Mango and Kiwi Salsa 438	*Leftover* Ground Turkey and Vegetable Stuffed Bell Peppers..............302 *Leftover* 1½ cups Roasted Vegetables................................79 *Leftover* ½ cup Basic Brown Rice........129	Mini Parfait (page 137) 204	1,484
Saturday	*Leftover* Egg and Avocado Burrito...........280 1 cup diced cantaloupe......60	*Leftover* Black Bean, Corn, and Chicken Sausage Bowl....338 1 medium apple ..95	*Leftover* Seafood à la Paella with Farro ....281 1 ounce dark chocolate (at least 75% dark).................160	*Leftover* Roasted Vegetable Soup with Parmesan Cheese 115	1,329
Sunday	¾ cup 2% Greek yogurt + 8 strawberries + 1 tablespoon chopped walnuts + 1 teaspoon honey 255	*Leftover* Black Bean, Corn, and Chicken Sausage Bowl....338 1 medium apple ..95	*Leftover* Ground Turkey and Vegetable Stuffed Bell Peppers..............302 *Leftover* 1½ cups Roasted Vegetables................................79 *Leftover* ½ cup Basic Brown Rice........129	25 grapes + 2 light string cheeses 190	1,388

Shopping List

PRODUCE

FRESH

- Apples, medium (5)
- Avocado, medium (1)
- Bell peppers, any color (5)
- Bell peppers, red (4)
- Berries (¾ cup)
- Brussels sprouts (2 cups)
- Carrot (1)
- Cantaloupe (1)
- Cauliflower, 1 head
- Celery (3 stalks)
- Cilantro (1 bunch)
- Cucumbers (2)
- Grapes (1 pound)
- Jalapeño (1)
- Lemon (1)
- Mangos (3)
- Mint (1 bunch)
- Onions, red (3)
- Onion, yellow (1)
- Onion, white (1)
- Strawberries (1 pound)
- Sungold kiwis (2)
- Yellow summer squash (2)
- Zucchini, green (2)

FROZEN

- Corn (1 cup)

EGGS AND DAIRY

- Eggs, large (6)
- Greek yogurt, plain, 2% (1¾ cups)
- Mozzarella cheese (4 ounces)

MEAT, POULTRY, AND SEAFOOD

- Chicken sausage links, reduced fat (4)
- Ground turkey, lean (1 pound)
- Mahi-mahi (1 pound)
- Scallops (4 ounces)
- Sole fish (8 ounces)
- Shrimp, large (20 to 25), peeled and deveined (1 pound)

PANTRY

DRIED HERBS AND SPICES

- Paprika, smoked
- Saffron

JARRED, BOTTLED, BAGGED, AND CANNED

- Black beans, 2 (15½-ounce) cans
- Broth, chicken or vegetable, 2 (32-ounce) cartons
- Corn tortillas, 6 (5-inch)
- Dark chocolate, 75% (3 ounces)
- Tomatoes, diced, 2 (14½-ounce) cans
- Tortillas, flour, high-fiber, 4 (7-inch)
- Whole-kernel corn, 1 (15½-ounce) can

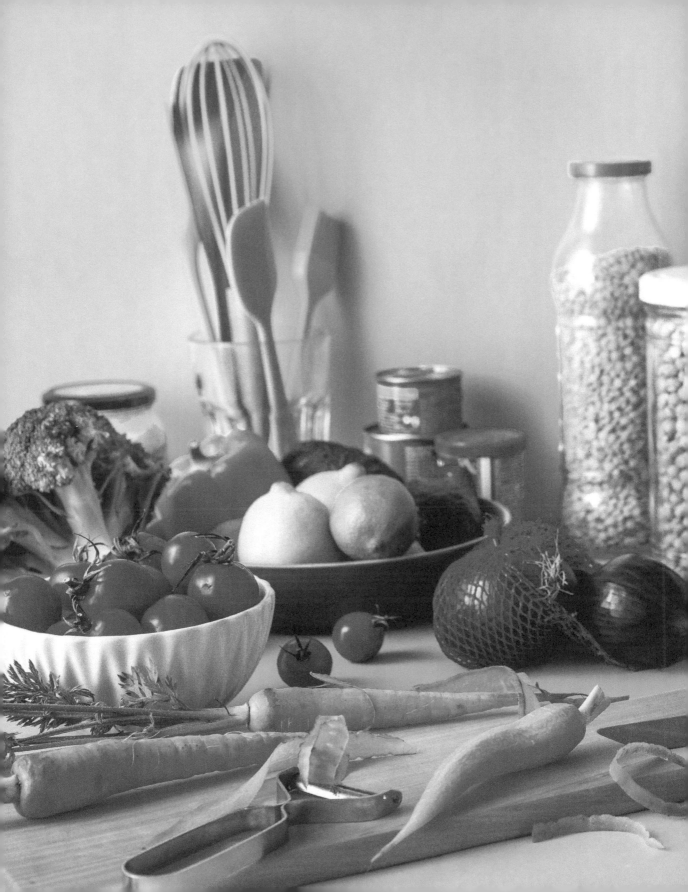

LOW-CALORIE RECIPES

In this section of the book, we finally get to the recipes you'll be enjoying over the next 4 weeks and beyond. The majority of the breakfasts, lunches, and dinners are less than 400 calories, and nearly all of the snacks and desserts are less than 250 calories. The recipes in chapter 8 (page 147) offer a low-calorie twist on commonly used dressings, sauces, and more that might not necessarily fit into a healthy low-calorie meal plan otherwise. You'll be using these food items throughout the book to enhance your meals and snacks.

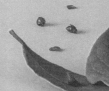

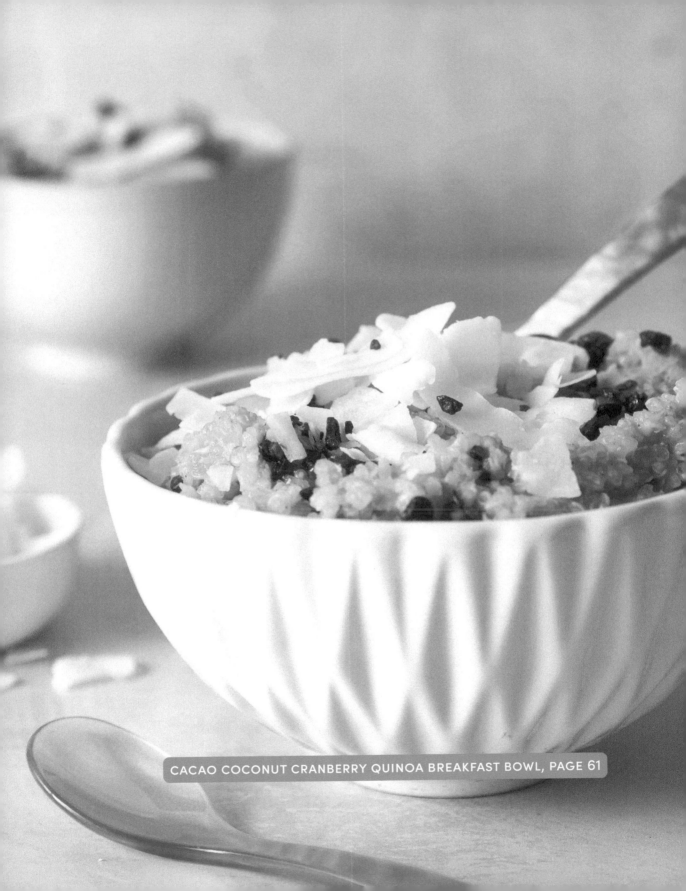

CACAO COCONUT CRANBERRY QUINOA BREAKFAST BOWL, PAGE 61

CHAPTER FOUR

BREAKFASTS

Warm Apple-Spiced Smoothie 54

Orange Delight Smoothie 55

Berry Mango Bliss Smoothie 56

Creamy Green Smoothie 57

Superfood Parfait 58

Spice-Infused Oatmeal 59

High-Protein Overnight Oats 60

Cacao Coconut Cranberry Quinoa Breakfast Bowl 61

Umami Scrambled Eggs 62

California-Style Scrambled Eggs 63

Sun-Dried Tomato and Vegetable Frittata 64

Crustless Egg and Spinach Quiches 66

Banana Cacao Oat Pancakes 67

Egg, Cheese, and Ham English Muffins 68

Egg and Avocado Burritos 70

Dried Fruit and Chia High-Protein Muffins 72

Butternut Squash Walnut Bread 74

Warm Apple-Spiced Smoothie

Vegetarian	Prep time: 5 minutes / Cook time: 1 minute / Serves: 1

Cinnamon combined with the natural sweetness of applesauce gives a nice balance to this smoothie. The addition of warm milk makes this treat perfect for chilly mornings. Look for a protein powder with at least 20 grams of protein and 2 grams or less of sugar per scoop.

1 cup 1% milk

¼ cup quick 1-minute oats

½ cup unsweetened applesauce

¼ teaspoon ground cinnamon

1 scoop vanilla protein powder

1. In a glass, warm the milk in the microwave for 1 minute.

2. Pour the milk into a high-speed blender, then add the remaining ingredients.

3. Blend until smooth. Pour into the same glass and enjoy.

Make it easier: You can enjoy this smoothie at room temperature or cold—just skip step 1.

Per serving: **Calories:** 299; **Fat:** 5g; **Carbohydrates:** 29g; Fiber: 3g; Sugar: 14g; Protein: 35g; Sodium: 347mg

Orange Delight Smoothie

Gluten-Free Vegetarian	Prep time: 10 minutes Serves: 1

Smoothies don't always have to be green! In order to get a wide variety of nutrients, it's beneficial to consume all colors of fruits and vegetables, so today, mix things up with this nutritious and refreshing orange smoothie.

1½ cups water

½ cup sliced carrots

½ orange, peeled

1 cup cubed cantaloupe

1 tablespoon chia seeds

¼ teaspoon ground cinnamon

1 scoop vanilla protein powder

1. Pour the water into a high-speed blender, then add the remaining ingredients.

2. Blend until smooth, pour into a tall glass, and enjoy.

Make it easier: You can make this smoothie the night before and refrigerate it in a sealed container for breakfast to go the next morning. The chia seeds will thicken the smoothie, so you can either add a bit more water the next day and shake, or add the chia seeds right before you drink the smoothie.

Per serving: Calories: 282; Fat: 4.5g; Carbohydrates: 34g; Fiber: 9.5g; Sugar: 22g; Protein: 28g; Sodium: 311mg

Berry Mango Bliss Smoothie

Gluten-Free Vegetarian	Prep time: 10 minutes Serves: 1

If you're into tropical fruits, this is the smoothie for you. The mango is a good source of vitamin C as well as antioxidants and phytonutrients. Also, as you'll discover, there are sneaky vegetables in this smoothie that you won't even be able to taste.

1 cup water

1 cup strawberries

1 cup peeled and coarsely chopped cucumber

1 cup coarsely chopped yellow zucchini

¾ cup coarsely chopped mango

1 tablespoon chia seeds

1 tablespoon lemon juice

2 mint leaves

1 scoop vanilla protein powder

1. Pour the water into a high-speed blender, then add the remaining ingredients.

2. Blend until smooth, pour into a tall glass, and enjoy.

Make it easier: You can also use thawed frozen mango for convenience.

Per serving: Calories: 332; Fat: 6g; Carbohydrates: 45g; Fiber: 12g; Sugar: 30g; Protein: 30g; Sodium: 257mg

Creamy Green Smoothie

Gluten-Free Vegetarian	Prep time: 10 minutes Serves: 1

Avocado provides a rich, creamy consistency in this smoothie. Fun fact: Adding fat (like avocado) to smoothies is an important step for absorbing fat-soluble vitamins from other fruits and vegetables. I use vanilla protein powder, but you can use any flavor you like.

1½ cups water

2 cups spinach

1 cup cubed pineapple

1 cup sliced cucumber

2 tablespoons chopped fresh parsley

½-inch knob peeled ginger

⅓ medium avocado, peeled and pitted

1 tablespoon lemon juice

1 scoop protein powder

1. Pour the water into a high-speed blender, then add the remaining ingredients.

2. Blend until smooth, pour into a tall glass, and enjoy.

Make it easier: You can use the same amount of frozen spinach and pineapple instead of fresh.

Per serving: Calories: 315; Fat: 8.5g; Carbohydrates: 36g; Fiber: 9g; Sugar: 19g; Protein: 28g; Sodium: 300mg

Superfood Parfait

Gluten-Free Vegetarian	Prep time: 5 minutes Serves: 1

This parfait is delicious, and it's full of superfoods. Cacao nibs are small pieces from the cacao seed that contain zero sugar and have been shown to curb cravings while you're on your weight loss journey.

1 cup plain 2% Greek yogurt

¾ cup frozen mixed berries, thawed

1 tablespoon crushed walnuts

1 tablespoon cacao nibs

1 teaspoon chia seeds

2 tablespoons Mixed Berries Sweet Sauce (page 158)

In a small serving bowl or jar with a lid, top the yogurt with the remaining ingredients.

Swap or substitute: If you don't have the sweet sauce made, you can use low-sugar or no-sugar-added jam.

Per serving: Calories: 368; Fat: 16g; Carbohydrates: 33g; Fiber: 8.5g; Sugar: 21g; Protein: 27g; Sodium: 84mg

Spice-Infused Oatmeal

Vegetarian	**Prep time:** 5 minutes / **Cook time:** 10 minutes / **Serves:** 4

This oatmeal is prepared the same way I had it growing up in Peru. In Latin America, we love to infuse our desserts and hot breakfast cereals with cinnamon and cloves. I hope you enjoy this new and easy way to make oatmeal.

2½ cups water

4 cloves

2 cinnamon sticks

2 cups quick 1-minute oats

4 tablespoons raisins

¼ teaspoon sea salt

2 cups 1% milk

Ground cinnamon

1. In a 4-quart pot, bring the water, cloves, and cinnamon sticks to a rolling boil and cook for 3 minutes.

2. Add the oats, raisins, and sea salt, reduce heat to low, and simmer for 2 minutes.

3. Add the milk and simmer, stirring frequently, for an additional 2 minutes, until thickened.

4. Spoon the oatmeal evenly into 4 bowls, sprinkle with ground cinnamon, and enjoy warm. Store leftover oatmeal in a sealed container in the refrigerator for up to 4 days.

Bulk it up: Top with a cup of berries of your choice before enjoying.

Per serving (1 cup): Calories: 232; Fat: 4g; Carbohydrates: 41g; Fiber: 4.5g; Sugar: 13g; Protein: 9g; Sodium: 55mg

High-Protein Overnight Oats

Vegetarian	Prep time: 10 minutes, plus 4 to 8 hours to chill / Serves: 4

These overnight oats can make either a filling breakfast or a quick and healthy snack. The soluble fiber from the oats will help keep you full until your next meal and is also good for your heart. Use your preferred milk here, as well as your favorite frozen berries or berry mix.

1 cup quick 1-minute oats

2 cups plain
  2% Greek yogurt

2 cups frozen berries

2 cups 1% milk

1 tablespoon ground
  cinnamon

¼ teaspoon sea salt

1. Equally divide the ingredients between 4 (12-ounce) lidded jars.

2. Using a spoon, stir the ingredients until fully incorporated.

3. Seal the jars and allow them to sit for at least 4 hours or up to overnight in the refrigerator until the oats have thickened, then enjoy.

> **Store it:** Make several jars in advance for an easy grab-and-go breakfast or snack. Store in sealed containers in the refrigerator for up to 4 days.

Per serving (1 jar): **Calories: 246**; Fat: 5.5g; Carbohydrates: 33g; Fiber: 4g; Sugar: 16g; Protein: 19g; Sodium: 241mg

Cacao Coconut Cranberry Quinoa Breakfast Bowl

Gluten-Free Vegetarian	Prep time: 5 minutes / Cook time: 20 minutes / Serves: 4

For those looking for a substitute for sugary cereals, here's a bowl with some superfood sweetness. Quinoa is a great base for a hot breakfast cereal, and it provides high fiber and protein, two nutrients pivotal to any weight loss plan.

2 cups water

4 cloves

2 cinnamon sticks

1 cup dry quinoa

Pinch sea salt

1 cup 1% milk

2 tablespoons unsweetened dried cranberries

1 tablespoon unsweetened shredded coconut

1 tablespoon cacao nibs

Ground cinnamon

1. In a 4-quart pot, bring the water, cloves, and cinnamon sticks to a rolling boil and cook for 3 minutes.

2. Add the quinoa and salt, reduce heat to medium, and cook, stirring occasionally, for 10 minutes, or until the quinoa starts to soften.

3. Add the milk, reduce heat to medium-low, and cook, stirring frequently, for an additional 5 minutes.

4. Add the cranberries, coconut, and cacao nibs and mix well.

5. Spoon evenly into 4 bowls and sprinkle with cinnamon. Serve warm.

Store it: Store leftovers in a sealed container in the refrigerator for up to 4 days.

Per serving (¾ cup): Calories: 216; Fat: 5g; Carbohydrates: 34g; Fiber: 4g; Sugar: 6.5g; Protein: 8g; Sodium: 64mg

Umami Scrambled Eggs

Gluten-Free Vegetarian	Prep time: 5 minutes / Cook time: 5 minutes / Serves: 4

These scrambled eggs will activate your fifth taste receptor, the umami receptor. Monosodium glutamate (MSG) is umami. MSG has had a bad reputation that has now been debunked. This lower-sodium salt substitute adds a punch of flavor to food and is completely safe to use based on the latest research (see Resources, page 161).

Nonstick cooking spray

5 scallions, green and white parts, sliced

1 cup sliced baby bella mushrooms

8 large eggs

¼ cup shredded Parmesan cheese

1 tablespoon tomato paste

½ teaspoon umami seasoning (MSG)

⅛ teaspoon sea salt

1. In a large nonstick skillet sprayed with cooking spray, cook the scallions and mushrooms over medium heat, stirring occasionally, for 3 minutes.

2. In a medium bowl, whisk together the eggs, cheese, tomato paste, umami seasoning, and sea salt until well combined.

3. Pour the egg mixture into the skillet with the vegetables. Move the eggs around gently with a wooden spoon and cook over medium-low heat for 2 to 3 minutes, or until the eggs are cooked through.

4. Divide the mixture between 4 plates and serve warm. Store leftovers in a sealed container in the refrigerator for up to 3 days.

Bulk it up: Enjoy these eggs with some whole-grain toast or a cup of fresh fruit.

Per serving (¾ cup): **Calories:** 188; Fat: 12g; Carbohydrates: 4g; Fiber: 1g; Sugar: 1.5g; Protein: 15g; Sodium: 476mg

California-Style Scrambled Eggs

Dairy-Free Gluten-Free Vegetarian	**Prep time:** 5 minutes **Cook time:** 5 minutes **Serves:** 1

If there's a fruit that's a favorite in California, it's avocados! The creamy texture of avocado and the fresh flavor of tomatoes and cilantro go wonderfully with these scrambled eggs.

Nonstick cooking spray

3 large eggs

¼ cup halved cherry tomatoes

1 tablespoon chopped cilantro

¼ teaspoon sea salt

⅓ medium avocado, peeled, pitted, and cubed

1. Heat a medium skillet over medium heat and spray it with cooking spray.

2. In a medium bowl, whisk together the eggs, tomatoes, cilantro, and salt until well combined.

3. Pour the egg mixture into the skillet. Move the eggs around gently with a wooden spoon. After 1½ minutes, add the avocado. Mix well and serve warm.

Per serving: Calories: 327; Fat: 26g; Carbohydrates: 6g; Fiber: 3.5g; Sugar: 1.5g; Protein: 20g; Sodium: 800mg

Sun-Dried Tomato and Vegetable Frittata

Dairy-Free Gluten-Free Vegetarian	Prep time: 10 minutes Cook time: 15 minutes Serves: 4

This isn't one of those recipes you can whip together on a busy workday morning, but it is definitely a savory, warm egg breakfast you'll want to use your weekend time to put together. Let me tell you, it's well worth the time you put in! I suggest using a frozen vegetable blend of carrots, corn, and green beans.

1 tablespoon extra-virgin olive oil

½ medium red onion, diced

1 medium orange bell pepper, diced

3 ounces sun-dried tomatoes, not in oil, diced

6 scallions, green and white parts, sliced

2 cups mixed frozen vegetables, thawed

8 large eggs

½ teaspoon dried thyme

½ teaspoon sea salt

¼ teaspoon freshly ground black pepper

1. In a large nonstick skillet, heat the oil over medium heat for 1 minute.

2. In the skillet, cook the red onion, bell pepper, and sun-dried tomatoes for 4 minutes, stirring occasionally.

3. Add the scallions and thawed vegetables and cook for another 2 minutes, stirring occasionally.

4. In a medium bowl, crack the eggs; add the thyme, salt, and pepper; and whisk well.

5. Pour the egg mixture into the skillet and mix all the ingredients well. Cover, reduce heat to medium-low, and cook for about 10 minutes, or until the frittata becomes puffy and firm.

6. Cut the frittata into 4 wedges and enjoy warm. Store leftovers in a sealed container in the refrigerator for up to 4 days.

Make it easier: Quickly thaw the vegetables by placing them in a sieve or colander and running warm water over them for up to a minute.

Per serving (1 wedge): **Calories:** 303; Fat: 14g; Carbohydrates: 28g; Fiber: 6g; Sugar: 14g; Protein: 18g; Sodium: 479mg

Crustless Egg and Spinach Quiches

Gluten-Free Vegetarian	Prep time: 5 minutes / Cook time: 25 minutes / Serves: 4

Eggs are an excellent low-calorie source of protein and healthy fat. These are two macronutrients that help keep you full and satiated, making this the ideal breakfast food to power you through your mornings. Prepare these quiches on the weekend and store them for a quick grab-and-go breakfast during your busy week.

Nonstick cooking spray

3 cups frozen chopped spinach

12 large eggs

3 ounces feta cheese

¼ teaspoon freshly ground black pepper

Pinch sea salt

1. Preheat the oven to 350°F. Mist 12 cups of a muffin tin with cooking spray and set aside.

2. In a large microwave-safe bowl, defrost the chopped spinach in the microwave for about 2 minutes. Squeeze out the excess liquid from the spinach.

3. In the bowl with the spinach, crack the eggs and stir to incorporate. Add the feta cheese, pepper, and salt and mix well.

4. Spoon the mixture evenly into the muffin cups, up to ½ inch from the top. Bake for 20 to 25 minutes, or until puffed and lightly browned.

5. Enjoy immediately or cool and store leftovers in a sealed container in the refrigerator for up to 4 days.

> **Make it easier:** Use foil or paper muffin liners for easy cleanup.

Per serving (3 quiches): Calories: 335; Fat: 24g; Carbohydrates: 7g; Fiber: 3.5g; Sugar: 2g; Protein: 26g; Sodium: 529mg

Banana Cacao Oat Pancakes

Vegetarian	**Prep time:** 10 minutes / **Cook time:** 15 minutes / **Serves:** 4

These pancakes are a must-try! Low-calorie, satisfying, and a nutrition powerhouse, this is not just a dish for your weight loss plan, but a tasty meal you can share with your entire family. They will love you for this breakfast.

2 medium bananas

2 large eggs

½ cup plain
  2% Greek yogurt

½ cup 1% milk

1 cup quick 1-minute oats

1 tablespoon canola oil

2 teaspoons
  baking powder

1 teaspoon vanilla extract

½ teaspoon ground
  cinnamon

¼ teaspoon sea salt

1 tablespoon cacao nibs

Nonstick cooking spray

½ cup Mixed Berries
  Sweet Sauce (page 158)

1. In a high-speed blender, combine the bananas, eggs, yogurt, milk, oats, oil, baking powder, vanilla, cinnamon, and salt. Blend on high until completely smooth, about 30 seconds.

2. Add the cacao nibs to the batter and mix well with a spatula or spoon.

3. Coat a griddle or large nonstick skillet with cooking spray and heat over medium-low heat.

4. Once the pan is hot, add ⅓ cup of batter to the skillet for each pancake. Cook for 3 minutes or until the pancakes slightly puff up and bubble along the edges. Flip and cook for 1 to 2 minutes more.

5. Remove the pancakes and place them on a cooling rack or plate. Repeat until you've used up the batter. Top each pancake with 1 tablespoon of berry sauce and serve warm.

Store it: Store leftover pancakes in a sealed container in the refrigerator for up to 3 days.

Per serving (2 pancakes + 2 tablespoons sauce): Calories: 289; Fat: 13g; Carbohydrates: 36g; Fiber: 5g; Sugar: 14g; Protein: 11g; Sodium: 205mg

Egg, Cheese, and Ham English Muffins

Prep time: 15 minutes / **Cook time:** 5 minutes / **Serves:** 4

For fast-food breakfast lovers, this easy recipe will give you those delicious flavors without all the excess calories, but enough protein and whole grains to keep you going all morning. This calls for Canadian bacon, which is more like ham than other bacon. Just be sure to use "lite" cheese that is 4 grams of fat or less per slice.

4 large eggs

2 ounces Canadian bacon, diced

½ teaspoon sea salt

¼ teaspoon freshly ground black pepper

Nonstick cooking spray

4 (1-ounce) slices Jarlsberg lite cheese

4 whole-grain English muffins

1. In a medium bowl, combine the eggs, bacon, salt, and pepper. Whisk well.

2. Heat a large nonstick skillet over medium heat, and place 4 (3-inch) biscuit molds on top of the skillet.

3. Pour the egg mixture evenly into the molds. Cover and cook until the egg mixture is set, 2 to 3 minutes. Using a spatula, remove each mold, and using oven mitts, remove the egg cakes by pushing each out with a spoon.

4. Meanwhile, if desired, warm your English muffins in a toaster or toaster oven, or microwave them on high for 20 seconds.

5. Place an egg cake on a halved English muffin and immediately add a slice of cheese on top. Top with the other half of the English muffin. Repeat with the remaining eggs, muffins, and cheese. Enjoy warm. Wrap leftovers in aluminum foil and store in the refrigerator for up to 4 days.

Make it easier: If you don't have biscuit molds, simply cook the eggs and ham like a scramble and divide the scramble between the 4 muffins, then add the cheese.

Per serving (1 sandwich): **Calories:** 298; Fat: 12g; Carbohydrates: 27g; Fiber: 2.5g; Sugar: 1g; Protein: 23g; Sodium: 840mg

Egg and Avocado Burritos

Vegetarian	Prep time: 5 minutes / Cook time: 5 minutes / Serves: 4

Who doesn't like a good breakfast burrito? This low-calorie but nutritious burrito is sure to spice up your morning routine. When choosing tortillas, look for a brand with no more than 80 calories and at least 7 grams of fiber per tortilla.

Nonstick cooking spray

4 large eggs

½ cup shredded part-skim mozzarella cheese

¼ teaspoon sea salt

¼ teaspoon freshly ground black pepper

4 (7-inch) light high-fiber flour tortillas

1 medium avocado, peeled, pitted, and sliced

1. Spray a large nonstick skillet with cooking spray and heat over medium-low heat.

2. In a medium bowl, whisk together the eggs, mozzarella, salt, and pepper until well combined.

3. Pour the eggs into the skillet and move them around gently with a wooden spoon. Cook for 2 to 3 minutes or until the eggs are set.

4. Equally divide the egg mixture across the bottom half of 4 tortillas. Place ¼ of the avocado on top of each egg mixture.

5. Fold the bottom of the tortilla up and over the filling, and pull the filling back toward the bottom third of the tortilla. Make two folds on either side of the large fold so all the egg is contained inside the fold.

6. Roll the tortilla up, using the tips of your fingers to tuck and press the filling into a tight cylinder. Repeat with the remaining tortillas and eggs. Serve warm or wrap the burritos in aluminum foil and store in the refrigerator for up to 4 days.

Swap or substitute: If you want more flavor, feel free to top these burritos with store-bought salsa. Tomato-based green and red salsas are usually lower in calories. Look for those with 10 or fewer calories per serving.

Per serving (1 burrito): **Calories:** 280; Fat: 16g; Carbohydrates: 28g; Fiber: 10g; Sugar: 3.5g; Protein: 15g; Sodium: 633mg

Dried Fruit and Chia High-Protein Muffins

Vegetarian	**Prep time:** 15 minutes / **Cook time:** 20 minutes / **Serves:** 12

Traditional baked goods are usually full of sugar and fat and tend to be anything but "low-calorie." These muffins are a great replacement for store-bought bakery sweets without the high-calorie price tag. They also make a wonderful grab-and-go breakfast or snack.

Nonstick cooking spray

1 cup all-purpose flour

1 cup quick 1-minute oats

2 scoops vanilla
   protein powder

2 tablespoons chia seeds

1 teaspoon baking soda

1 teaspoon baking powder

1 teaspoon sea salt

2 medium ripe
   bananas, mashed

½ cup plain 2%
   Greek yogurt

½ cup 1% milk

2 large eggs

2 tablespoons canola oil

1 teaspoon vanilla extract

5 dried prunes,
   finely chopped

5 dried apricots,
   finely chopped

1. Preheat the oven to 350°F. Line 12 cups of a muffin tin with paper liners and spray them with cooking spray. Set aside.

2. In a large bowl, whisk the flour, oats, protein powder, chia seeds, baking soda, baking powder, and salt until well blended. Set aside.

3. In a medium bowl, whisk together the bananas, yogurt, milk, eggs, oil, and vanilla until well combined.

4. Pour the wet ingredients into the dry ingredients and stir until just combined. Stir in the chopped prunes and apricots.

5. Spoon the batter into the muffin cups and bake for 20 minutes, or until a toothpick inserted in the center of a muffin comes out clean.

6. Serve warm. Store leftovers in a sealed container in the refrigerator for up to 7 days.

Swap or substitute: You can replace the prunes and apricots with the same quantity of any dried fruit.

Per serving (1 muffin): **Calories: 171;** Fat: 6.5g; Carbohydrates: 23g; Fiber: 3g; Sugar: 6g; Protein: 7g; Sodium: 347mg

Butternut Squash Walnut Bread

Vegetarian	**Prep time:** 10 minutes / **Cook time:** 1 hour 15 minutes / **Serves:** 10

Who would have thought you could contribute to your daily vegetable intake with a delicious and low-calorie bread? The vegetables give this savory bread nice texture, and the zero-calorie monk fruit sweetener gives it just a touch of sweetness.

3 cups (14½ ounces) peeled and cubed butternut squash

Nonstick cooking spray

1½ cups all-purpose flour

1½ cups quick 1-minute oats

½ cup monk fruit sweetener or stevia

1 teaspoon ground cinnamon

1 teaspoon baking powder

1 teaspoon baking soda

1 teaspoon sea salt

½ cup 1% milk

2 large eggs

2 tablespoons canola oil

2 teaspoons vanilla extract

½ cup chopped walnuts

1. In a large pot, cover the squash with cold water. Bring to a boil over high heat and cook for 15 minutes or until soft. Drain the water and transfer the squash to a large bowl. Using a fork, mash the squash. Let cool for about 10 minutes.

2. Meanwhile, preheat the oven to 350°F. Spray a 9-inch loaf pan with nonstick spray and set aside.

3. In a medium bowl, stir together the flour, oats, monk fruit sweetener, cinnamon, baking powder, baking soda, and salt until well mixed. Set aside.

4. When the squash is cooled, add the milk, eggs, oil, and vanilla and mix until well blended.

5. Gently whisk the dry ingredients into the wet ingredients until just combined. Fold in the walnuts.

6. Spoon the batter into the prepared loaf pan and place in the oven on the middle rack. Bake for 60 minutes or until golden brown and a toothpick inserted in the center comes out clean.

7. Cut into 10 slices and serve warm. Store leftovers in a sealed container in the refrigerator for up to 5 days.

Store it: Slice and freeze leftover bread in a sealed zip-top bag for up to 3 months. Reheat individual slices in an oven or toaster.

Per serving (1 slice): **Calories:** 225; Fat: 9.5g; Carbohydrates: 30g; Fiber: 3g; Sugar: 3g; Protein: 6g; Sodium: 380mg

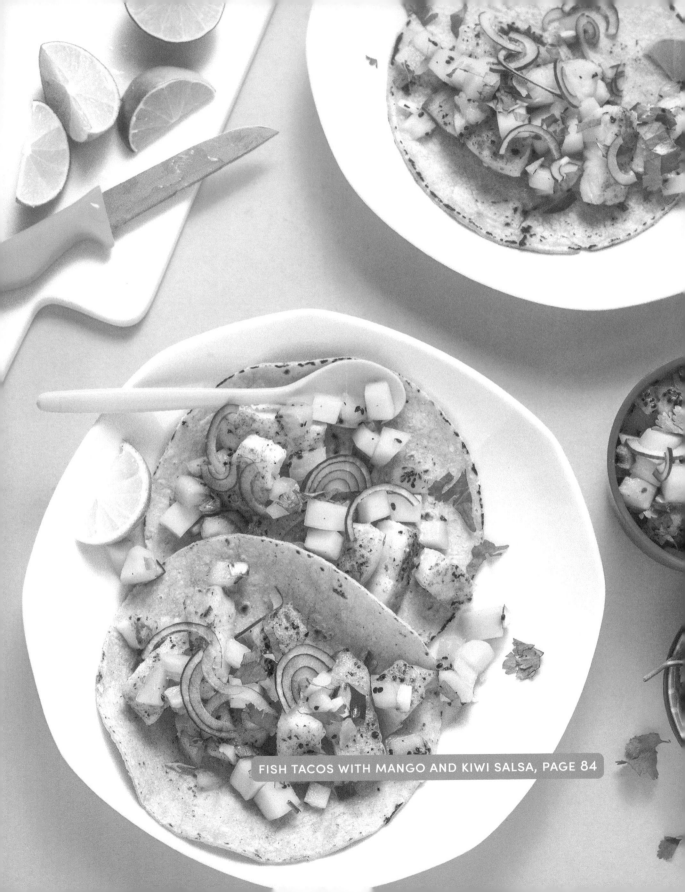

FISH TACOS WITH MANGO AND KIWI SALSA, PAGE 84

CHAPTER FIVE

LUNCHES

Avocado, Tomato, and Poached Egg Toast 78

Roast Beef and Cheese Panini 79

Turkey Spinach Roll 80

Curried Chicken Pita Wraps 81

Chicken Apple Salad 82

Citrus Quinoa Avocado Salad with Roasted Chicken 83

Fish Tacos with Mango and Kiwi Salsa 84

Ground Pork Endive Cups 85

Caramelized Onions and Spinach with
Glazed Balsamic Salmon 87

Chicken Cilantro Patties 89

Salmon Cakes Salad 90

Chicken and Potato Salad with Yogurt Dressing 92

Tomato Chickpea Soup 93

Turkey Meatball Quinoa Soup 94

Light Farfalle and Cheese with Cauliflower 96

Black Bean, Corn, and Chicken Sausage Bowl 98

Chicken Pomodoro Farro Bowl 99

Shrimp and Vegetable Wild Rice Bowl 100

Avocado, Tomato, and Poached Egg Toast

Dairy-Free Vegetarian	Prep time: 5 minutes / Cook time: 5 minutes / Serves: 1

Avocado toast has become a trendy dish. However, when I lived in Peru, we used to enjoy a sandwich with avocado, tomato, and egg on it (called "the Triple") all the time. That dish inspired this one. I hope you enjoy it as much as I did in my childhood.

1 large egg

Red wine vinegar

1 slice whole-grain bread, toasted

¼ medium avocado, peeled, pitted, and sliced

3 slices tomato

1. Crack the egg into a small bowl.

2. In a 10-inch skillet, bring 2 inches of water to a simmer over medium heat. Add a drop of vinegar.

3. With a spatula, stir the water to create a gentle whirlpool to help the egg white wrap around the yolk. Tip the egg into the pan. The yolk should follow the white.

4. Cook for 3 to 4 minutes, or until the egg white is opaque. The yolk will be runny (see tip). Meanwhile, toast the bread to desired doneness.

5. With a slotted spoon, lift the egg out of the pan. Set on a paper towel to dry.

6. Spread the avocado on the toast, then layer on the tomatoes. Place the poached egg on top and enjoy.

> **Swap or substitute:** Not everyone likes a runny egg, so if you would like to hard-boil or fry your egg instead, feel free.

Per serving: **Calories: 229**; Fat: 11g; Carbohydrates: 23g; Fiber: 5g; Sugar: 4g; Protein: 12g; Sodium: 267mg

Roast Beef and Cheese Panini

Prep time: 10 minutes / **Cook time:** 10 minutes / **Serves:** 2

I find that warming a sandwich makes it more filling. Melted cheese and flavorful roast beef combine in a satisfyingly mouthwatering sandwich you can enjoy for lunch or dinner. Look for a bread that's no more than 70 calories a slice.

1 medium tomato

⅛ teaspoon sea salt

¼ teaspoon freshly ground black pepper

1 teaspoon extra-virgin olive oil

4 slices light whole-grain bread

4 (1-ounce) slices deli-sliced roast beef

2 (1-ounce) slices Jarlsberg lite cheese

8 basil leaves

Nonstick cooking spray

1. Using a box grater or a hand grater, grate the tomato into a small bowl. Add the salt, pepper, and oil. Mix well, then spread the tomato mixture on top of the 4 bread slices.

2. Add 2 slices of roast beef on top of one slice of bread and the other 2 slices on top of another slice of bread. Then do the same with the cheese. Add 4 basil leaves on top and place the remaining bread slices on top of each sandwich.

3. Heat a large skillet over medium-low heat and spray it with cooking spray. Place the sandwiches in the skillet. Use a lid to press the sandwiches down. Cook on each side, pressing down, for 4 minutes. Serve warm.

Store it: Since this recipe makes two sandwiches, you can wrap the second one in aluminum foil and store it in the refrigerator for up to 3 days. When you're ready to eat it, place the sandwich without the foil in a preheated 250°F oven for 3 to 5 minutes. (Microwaving sandwiches can make the bread chewy and tough.)

Per serving (1 sandwich): Calories: 299; Fat: 13g; Carbohydrates: 16g; Fiber: 4g; Sugar: 3.5g; Protein: 28g; Sodium: 459mg

Turkey Spinach Roll

Prep time: 10 minutes / **Serves:** 1

Lunch doesn't have to be complicated! This recipe is for those super busy days when you need to throw something together quick. Don't worry though, it's not short on flavor—it's a tasty, satisfying lunch in a flash.

1 tablespoon avocado oil mayonnaise

1 (10-by-8-inch) whole-grain lavash bread

½ cup packed fresh spinach

½ cup shredded carrots

4 ounces deli-sliced turkey breast

1 (1-ounce) slice Jarlsberg lite cheese

1. Spread the mayonnaise over the lavash bread to about 1 inch from the edges.

2. Place the spinach and carrots over ⅓ of the bread and top with the turkey and cheese.

3. Starting at the short end, roll the bread into a wrap and cut in half. Enjoy.

Store it: You can make multiple rolls at once, wrap them in aluminum foil, and store them in the refrigerator for up to 2 days for a nice grab-and-go lunch.

Per serving: Calories: 398; Fat: 20g; Carbohydrates: 21g; Fiber: 9g; Sugar: 5g; Protein: 37g; Sodium: 1,215mg

Curried Chicken Pita Wraps

Prep time: 10 minutes / **Serves:** 4

If you're in the mood to try some flavors that are maybe not so familiar, here's a different take on chicken salad. The addition of raisins and curry creates a flavor that is out of this world, and the cashews deliver satisfying crunch. The avocado oil mayonnaise used has 60 calories with 7 grams of fat per tablespoon.

12 ounces Roasted Chicken, diced (page 148) or store-bought rotisserie chicken

2 (12-inch) celery stalks, chopped

5 scallions, green and white parts, chopped

½ cup plain 2% Greek yogurt

¼ cup raisins

¼ cup salted cashews

2 tablespoons avocado oil mayonnaise

1½ tablespoons curry powder

1 tablespoon lemon juice

½ teaspoon crushed ginger

¼ teaspoon sea salt

¼ teaspoon freshly ground black pepper

4 (6½-inch) whole-grain pitas

1. In a large bowl, combine the chicken, celery, scallions, yogurt, raisins, cashews, mayonnaise, curry powder, lemon juice, ginger, salt, and pepper and mix well to incorporate.

2. Cut a pita in half. Use a ¾-cup measuring cup to scoop out salad, and divide that between the two pita halves. Repeat for all the pitas.

Swap or substitute: Instead of pita, you can put this on leafy greens and enjoy it as a salad. Or open a can of garbanzo beans and enjoy ½ cup to 1 cup on the side.

Per serving (2 salad-filled pita halves): Calories: 454; Fat: 16g; Carbohydrates: 48g; Fiber: 6.5g; Sugar: 10g; Protein: 34g; Sodium: 1,241mg

Chicken Apple Salad

Gluten-Free	Prep time: 15 minutes / Serves: 4

I have a confession to make: I got the idea to add apples to my chicken salad from Oprah, and I've never looked back! Apples are a sweet, crunchy addition to traditional chicken salad, and they can help you meet your daily fruit servings.

12 ounces finely diced Roasted Chicken (page 148), or rotisserie chicken

2 (12-inch) celery stalks, chopped

1 medium Jazz apple (or any other apple), diced

¼ cup thinly chopped red onion

2 tablespoons avocado oil mayonnaise

2½ tablespoons yellow mustard

¼ cup plain 2% Greek yogurt

¼ teaspoon sea salt

¼ teaspoon freshly ground black pepper

In a large bowl, mix all the ingredients until well combined.

Swap or substitute: You can do so many things with this salad depending on your mood, including having it on bread for a sandwich, spooned over leafy greens with some cherry tomatoes, or just as is. To bulk it up, use slices of whole-grain bread if your calories allow.

Per serving (1¼ cups): Calories: 227; Fat: 10g; Carbohydrates: 9g; Fiber: 2g; Sugar: 6g; Protein: 25g; Sodium: 979mg

Citrus Quinoa Avocado Salad with Roasted Chicken

Gluten-Free	Prep time: 10 minutes / Serves: 1

Most people are familiar with yellow quinoa, but this recipe uses red quinoa. All quinoas are prepared the same way regardless of the color, but different colors contain different phytonutrients. You can buy precooked quinoa either frozen or vacuum-packed and ready to use if you don't have time to prepare your own.

3 cups mixed greens

½ cup cooked Basic
   Flavorful Quinoa
   (page 151)

2 (12-inch) celery
   stalks, sliced

3 ounces diced Roasted
   Chicken (page 148), or
   rotisserie chicken

1 mandarin orange

¼ medium avocado,
   peeled, pitted,
   and sliced

⅓ cup shredded
   Parmesan cheese

¼ teaspoon sea salt

⅛ teaspoon freshly
   ground black pepper

Lemon juice

In a large bowl, mix all the ingredients until well combined.

Store it: This salad can be stored in a sealed container in the refrigerator for up to 3 days. Just squeeze lemon juice on the avocados so they don't brown too quickly.

Per serving: Calories: 503; Fat: 18g; Carbohydrates: 49g; Fiber: 11g; Sugar: 11g; Protein: 40g; Sodium: 2,010mg

Fish Tacos with Mango and Kiwi Salsa

Dairy-Free Gluten-Free	Prep time: 10 minutes / Cook time: 6 minutes / Serves: 3

You've got to try these fish tacos. The sweetness from the mango, the touch of sour from the kiwi, and the robust flavors of the onion and cilantro? Talk about an explosion of flavor. Mango and Sungold kiwi are both excellent sources of vitamin C. Tilapia can also be used as the protein in this recipe.

FOR THE SALSA

1 mango, peeled and diced

2 Sungold kiwis (or green kiwis), peeled and diced

1 jalapeño, seeded and diced

¼ cup chopped cilantro

¼ cup thinly sliced red onion

1 teaspoon extra-virgin olive oil

¼ teaspoon freshly ground black pepper

FOR THE FISH

1 pound mahi-mahi

½ teaspoon sea salt

¼ teaspoon freshly ground black pepper

1 teaspoon extra-virgin olive oil

6 (5-inch) corn tortillas

TO MAKE THE SALSA

1. In a large bowl, mix the mango, kiwis, jalapeño, cilantro, red onion, oil, and pepper until well combined.

2. Set aside.

TO MAKE THE FISH

3. On a plate, sprinkle the fish with salt and pepper on both sides.

4. In a large skillet over medium heat, heat the oil. In the skillet, panfry the fish for 3 minutes on each side, or until the fish is flaky and opaque inside.

5. To build your tacos, place about 2 ounces of fish on each tortilla and top with 2 tablespoons of salsa. Enjoy.

Make it easier: In a rush? You can use store-bought mango salsa. You can also use any extra salsa on top of the Roasted Chicken (page 148).

Per serving (2 tacos): Calories: 438; Fat: 18g; Carbohydrates: 41g; Fiber: 4g; Sugar: 22g; Protein: 30g; Sodium: 851mg

Ground Pork Endive Cups

Dairy-Free	**Prep time:** 10 minutes / **Cook time:** 10 minutes / **Serves:** 6

This is a great appetizer that beats your average store-bought veggie platter. Many people are familiar with butter lettuce cups, but the use of nice, crisp Belgian endive in this recipe might convert you for good.

2 teaspoons sesame oil

½ medium yellow
   onion, diced

1 pound extra-lean
   ground pork

1 tablespoon minced garlic

1 teaspoon minced ginger

½ cup basil, sliced

4 scallions, green and
   white parts, sliced

2 tablespoons
   reduced-sodium
   soy sauce

½ teaspoon sea salt

4 heads Belgian endive

1. In a medium skillet over medium heat, heat the oil. Add the yellow onion and sauté for about 2 minutes.

2. Add the pork, garlic, and ginger and sauté for 7 minutes or until the pork is no longer pink.

3. Stir in the basil, scallions, soy sauce, and salt, and cook for another 2 minutes.

4. Carefully remove the spears of the endive. Divide the pork mixture, placing 2 tablespoons of pork mixture into each spear. Serve warm.

Swap or substitute: Ideally, the pork used in this recipe should be 96% lean/4% fat. If you can't find a lean version, you can reduce the fat yourself: Just brown the pork, discard the grease, and lightly rinse the pork with hot water.

Per serving (½ cup pork + 2 endive spears): Calories: 124; Fat: 5g; Carbohydrates: 4g; Fiber: 1.5g; Sugar: 0.5g; Protein: 17g; Sodium: 242mg

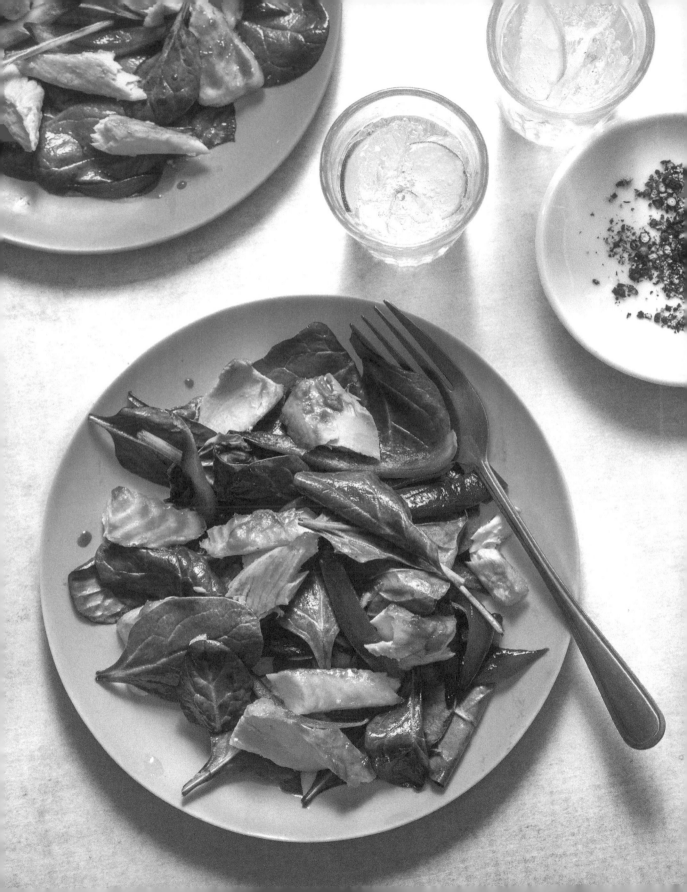

Caramelized Onions and Spinach with Glazed Balsamic Salmon

Dairy-Free Gluten-Free	Prep time: 10 minutes / Cook time: 10 minutes / Serves: 4

Who says salads need to be eaten cold? If you've never had a warm salad, I highly recommend starting with this one. The balsamic vinegar glaze is absolutely delicious and a must-have in the kitchen, as it adds a lot of flavor with minimal calories.

1 tablespoon extra-virgin olive oil

2 large red onions, cut into ½-inch slices

2 tablespoons balsamic vinegar glaze, store-bought or homemade (see tip)

1 teaspoon sea salt

12 cups baby spinach

12 ounces Glazed Balsamic Salmon (page 105)

1. Heat a medium skillet over medium heat for 1 minute. In the skillet, sauté the oil and onions for about 5 minutes, or until the onions become translucent. Leave the skillet covered except when stirring four times.

2. Add the balsamic vinegar glaze and salt and reduce heat to medium-low. Cover and cook for 2 minutes.

3. Add 3 cups of spinach at a time and cook, covered, for about 3 minutes until it wilts. Repeat three more times.

CONTINUED

4. Divide the caramelized onions and spinach into four portions, and top each with 3 ounces of baked salmon before serving. Store leftovers in a sealed container in the refrigerator for up to 4 days.

Make it easier: You can make your own glaze by simmering balsamic vinegar in a saucepan on medium-low until thickened, 10 to 15 minutes.

Per serving (1 cup vegetables + 3 ounces salmon): Calories: 306; Fat: 13g; Carbohydrates: 16g; Fiber: 5g; Sugar: 5.5g; Protein: 31g; Sodium: 1,062mg

Chicken Cilantro Patties

Dairy-Free Gluten-Free	Prep time: 10 minutes / Cook time: 10 minutes / Serves: 4

Enjoy these tasty, versatile patties over mixed greens with cherry tomatoes or, to bulk it up, make it a sandwich with two slices of whole-grain bread, sliced tomatoes, and lettuce leaves. You can find umami seasoning under the brand names Ajinomoto or Accent.

1 pound lean
  ground chicken

1 medium red bell pepper,
  finely diced

5 scallions, green and
  white parts, sliced

¼ cup finely chopped
  cilantro

½ teaspoon garlic powder

½ teaspoon umami
  seasoning (MSG)

½ teaspoon cumin

½ teaspoon sea salt

¼ teaspoon freshly
  ground black pepper

Nonstick cooking spray

1. In a large bowl, combine the chicken, bell pepper, scallions, cilantro, garlic powder, umami seasoning, cumin, salt, and pepper. Using your hands, mix all the ingredients well.

2. Divide the mixture into 4 patties and set them on a baking sheet or plate.

3. Spray a large skillet with cooking spray and heat it over medium heat. Place the patties in the skillet, cover, and cook for 5 minutes on one side. Flip the patties and cook, uncovered, for another 5 minutes.

4. Serve warm. Store leftovers in a sealed container in the refrigerator for up to 4 days.

Make it easier: You can batch cook these patties and store them in a zip-top bag in the freezer. Freeze for up to 6 months.

Per serving (1 patty): **Calories:** 151; **Fat:** 4.5g; **Carbohydrates:** 3g; **Fiber:** 1g; **Sugar:** 1.5g; **Protein:** 24g; **Sodium:** 393mg

Salmon Cakes Salad

Prep time: 10 minutes / **Cook time:** 10 minutes / **Serves:** 4

A lot of people think their salmon needs to come fresh-cut in a fillet. Salmon is one of those fishes you can buy canned and still enjoy its good flavor and nutrition. I always recommend having canned salmon in your pantry for recipes like this one.

FOR THE SALMON CAKES

3 (6-ounce) cans no-salt-added, skinless, boneless Alaskan pink salmon, drained

½ cup plain 2% Greek yogurt

¼ cup quick 1-minute oats

¼ cup finely diced red bell pepper

¼ cup chopped parsley

5 scallions, green and white parts, sliced

1 tablespoon lemon juice

2 teaspoons yellow mustard

1 teaspoon sea salt

½ teaspoon freshly ground black pepper

Nonstick cooking spray

TO MAKE THE SALMON CAKES

1. In a medium bowl, mix the salmon, yogurt, oats, bell pepper, parsley, scallions, lemon juice, mustard, salt, and pepper until well combined.

2. Divide the mixture into four cakes. With moistened hands, form the mixture into 4 round, flat patties.

3. Spray a large nonstick skillet with cooking spray and heat it over medium-low heat. Cook the salmon cakes for 3 to 4 minutes on each side, or until nicely browned.

FOR THE SALAD

12 cups baby arugula

2 cups cherry
tomatoes, halved

1 (15¼-ounce) can
whole-kernel
corn, drained

1 tablespoon lemon juice

TO MAKE THE SALAD

4. In a medium bowl, mix all the salad ingredients.

5. Divide the salad into four servings and place a
    salmon cake on top of each salad before serving.
    Store leftovers in a sealed container in the refriger-
    ator for up to 4 days.

> **Make it easier:** If you have biscuit molds, they
> can help shape your salmon cakes into the per-
> fect shape every time.

Per serving (1 salmon cake + ¼ salad): Calories: 271;
Fat: 7g; Carbohydrates: 25g; Fiber: 5g; Sugar: 10g;
Protein: 30g; Sodium: 1,300mg

Chicken and Potato Salad with Yogurt Dressing

Gluten-Free	Prep time: 10 minutes / Cook time: 30 minutes / Serves: 4

As a Peruvian, I am a potato lover! Many people think potatoes are not weight loss friendly. On the contrary, I have helped thousands of clients lose weight while still enjoying potatoes. To top it off, the cilantro-yogurt dressing gives this dish a nice Latin kick.

1½ pounds small tricolor potatoes

2 (7-inch) celery stalks, finely diced

¼ cup finely diced red onion

4 scallions, green and white parts, diced

¼ teaspoon sea salt

¾ cup Cilantro-Infused Yogurt Dressing (page 156)

12 ounces Roasted Chicken (page 148) or rotisserie chicken

1. In a large pot, cover the potatoes with cold water. Bring to a boil over high heat, reduce heat to low, and simmer for 20 minutes, or until soft. Drain the potatoes and set aside to cool. Once they are cool, cut them in half.

2. In a large bowl, stir together the celery, red onion, scallions, salt, and dressing. Add the potatoes and mix well to thoroughly coat the potatoes.

3. Divide between four bowls and top each with 3 ounces of chicken before serving.

Store it: Store leftovers in a sealed container in the refrigerator for up to 4 days.

Per serving (3 ounces chicken + ⅔ cup salad): Calories: 349; Fat: 12g; Carbohydrates: 32g; Fiber: 5.5g; Sugar: 4.5g; Protein: 29g; Sodium: 1,040mg

Tomato Chickpea Soup

Dairy-Free Gluten-Free	Prep time: 10 minutes / Cook time: 30 minutes / Serves: 4

Here's another easy recipe, a delicious and satiating soup that you can make in advance. It freezes for up to 6 months, so you can batch cook it for a convenient lunch or snack on busy days.

1 tablespoon extra-virgin olive oil

1 medium red onion, coarsely chopped

1 red bell pepper, chopped

1 (15-ounce) can artichoke hearts, in water, chopped

1 (14½-ounce) can diced tomatoes

1 (6-ounce) can tomato paste

1 cup low-sodium chicken broth

1 teaspoon smoked paprika

1 teaspoon sea salt

2 (15-ounce) cans chickpeas, drained and rinsed

¼ cup chopped fresh basil

1. In a 4-quart pot over medium-high heat, heat the oil. Add the onion, bell pepper, and artichokes and cook, stirring occasionally, for about 5 minutes.

2. Stir in the diced tomatoes, tomato paste, broth, paprika, and salt, and cook for about 5 minutes, stirring occasionally.

3. Transfer the mixture into a blender and carefully blend until smooth. Pour the purée back into the pot, cover, and simmer for 15 minutes over low heat, stirring a couple times.

4. Add the chickpeas and basil and simmer, covered, for another 5 minutes before serving. Store leftovers in a sealed container in the refrigerator for up to 4 days.

Bulk it up: You can add cooked shredded Roasted Chicken (page 148) or even pair this soup with the Roast Beef and Cheese Panini (page 79).

Per serving (1½ cups): Calories: 357; Fat: 6.5g; Carbohydrates: 60g; Fiber: 15g; Sugar: 16g; Protein: 16g; Sodium: 1,893mg

Turkey Meatball Quinoa Soup

Dairy-Free Gluten-Free	Prep time: 15 minutes / Cook time: 15 minutes / Serves: 4

Yellow quinoa is used in this recipe because it's softer than red, which makes it a perfect carbohydrate source to add to a soup. The ground turkey is a great lean protein that gives this soup nice body and boldness.

FOR THE MEATBALLS

1 pound lean
    ground turkey

½ medium red bell
    pepper, diced

¼ cup diced red onion

¾ cup Basic Flavorful
    Quinoa (page 151)

1 teaspoon sea salt

¼ teaspoon freshly
    ground black pepper

TO MAKE THE MEATBALLS

1. In a large bowl, mix together the ground turkey, bell pepper, onion, quinoa, salt, and pepper.

2. Divide the mixture into 12 portions (about ¼ cup each) and roll into meatballs about 2 inches in diameter. Place on a baking sheet or plate and set aside.

FOR THE SOUP

4 cups low-sodium
chicken broth

2 (7-inch) celery
stalks, sliced

2 (7-inch) carrots, sliced

1 (7-inch) zucchini, cubed

1 cup cooked Basic
Flavorful Quinoa
(page 151)

½ teaspoon umami
seasoning (MSG)

¼ teaspoon sea salt

¼ teaspoon freshly ground
black pepper

¼ cup cilantro leaves

TO MAKE THE SOUP

3. In a large 4-quart stockpot, bring the broth to a boil over high heat. Add the celery, carrots, and zucchini and simmer for 2 minutes over medium heat.

4. Carefully add the meatballs to the boiling broth and simmer for 8 minutes, or until the meatballs are cooked through and vegetables tender.

5. Stir in the quinoa and season the soup with umami seasoning, salt, and pepper. Serve warm, garnished with cilantro leaves. Store leftovers in a sealed container in the refrigerator for up to 4 days.

Make it easier: When making the meatballs, wet your hands before handling meat to keep it from sticking.

Per serving (1½ cups soup + 3 meatballs): Calories: 315; Fat: 10g; Carbohydrates: 27g; Fiber: 4g; Sugar: 5.5g; Protein: 29g; Sodium: 1,143mg

Light Farfalle and Cheese with Cauliflower

Vegetarian	Prep time: 10 minutes / Cook time: 30 minutes / Serves: 6

Mac and cheese is one of my favorite American side dishes—I fell in love with it when I came to this country. I wanted to come up with an idea on how to bring mac and cheese into low-calorie eating, and high-protein noodles were a key part of that. Cauliflower is also added for a dose of phytonutrients and low-calorie bulk.

8 ounces whole-grain protein-enriched farfalle pasta

3½ cups cauliflower florets, cut into small pieces

Nonstick cooking spray

1½ cups 1% milk

2 tablespoons cornstarch

1 teaspoon sea salt

¼ teaspoon freshly ground black pepper

1 cup shredded cheddar cheese

2 cups shredded part-skim mozzarella cheese

½ cup panko bread crumbs

1. Bring a 4-quart saucepan of water to a boil. Add the farfalle and cauliflower and cook for 8 to 9 minutes, stirring frequently. Drain and set aside.

2. Meanwhile, preheat the oven to 450°F. Spray a 9-by-13-inch baking dish with cooking spray and set aside.

3. In a 2-quart saucepan, combine the milk, cornstarch, salt, and pepper. Whisk until smooth. Place over medium heat and cook, stirring constantly, until the mixture boils and thickens, 2 to 3 minutes. Remove from heat. Stir in the cheddar and mozzarella and mix until almost melted.

4. Add the cooked pasta and cauliflower to the cheese mixture and mix well. Spoon into the prepared baking dish and evenly sprinkle with the panko bread crumbs. Bake for 20 to 25 minutes, or until golden on top.

5. Divide into six 4-inch squares and serve warm. Store leftovers in a sealed container in the refrigerator for up to 4 days.

Store it: This recipe freezes well if you're not planning on eating the whole thing right away. Freeze in a sealed container for up to 6 months.

Per serving (1 square): Calories: 408; Fat: 17g; Carbohydrates: 44g; Fiber: 1g; Sugar: 6.5g; Protein: 24g; Sodium: 954mg

Black Bean, Corn, and Chicken Sausage Bowl

Dairy-Free Gluten-Free	Prep time: 10 minutes / Cook time: 15 minutes / Serves: 4

Canned foods are very nutritious, convenient, and budget-friendly, and this tasty bowl makes good use of them. I always recommend keeping canned beans, corn, and tomatoes on hand in case you need to make something fast. When choosing a chicken sausage, choose a brand that has 6 grams of fat or less per link. You can also use vegetarian sausage.

2 teaspoons canola oil

4 reduced-fat chicken sausage links, sliced

1 medium red onion, diced

1 medium red bell pepper, diced

2 (12-inch) celery stalks, diced

1 cup frozen whole-kernel corn

1 teaspoon sea salt

¼ teaspoon freshly ground black pepper

2 (15½-ounce) cans black beans, drained and rinsed

1 (14½-ounce) can diced tomatoes

¼ cup chopped fresh cilantro

1. In a 4-quart pot over high heat, heat the oil and sauté the sausage for 4 minutes, stirring occasionally.

2. Add the onion, bell pepper, celery, corn, salt, and pepper. Reduce heat to medium, cover, and cook, stirring occasionally, for another 4 minutes, until the vegetables are soft.

3. Add the black beans and tomatoes and mix well. Cover and cook for 4 minutes, stirring occasionally.

4. Add the cilantro and mix well. Serve warm. Store leftovers in a sealed container in the refrigerator for up to 4 days.

Swap or substitute: If you can find canned or frozen roasted corn, use that for a boost in flavor.

Per serving (2 cups): **Calories: 338;** Fat: 5.5g; Carbohydrates: 55g; Fiber: 16g; Sugar: 7g; Protein: 19g; Sodium: 1,308mg

Chicken Pomodoro Farro Bowl

Dairy-Free	**Prep time:** 15 minutes / **Cook time:** 20 minutes / **Serves:** 6

Pomodoro is an Italian word that means "tomato." Tomato sauce is the base of this chicken stew that is easy and delicious, as well as a good source of lycopene. Lycopene, an antioxidant in tomatoes, is absorbed in the body 12 times better when tomatoes are cooked or canned when compared to raw.

1 tablespoon extra-virgin olive oil

1 large yellow onion, diced

2 (12-inch) celery stalks, chopped

4 (8-inch) carrots, sliced

1 tablespoon chopped garlic

1½ teaspoons sea salt

½ teaspoon freshly ground black pepper

1 cup low-sodium chicken broth

2 pounds boneless, skinless chicken breast

1 (14.5-ounce) can diced tomatoes

1 (6-ounce) can tomato paste

2 cups frozen peas

Basic Farro (page 149)

1. In a 4-quart pot over medium heat, heat the oil and sauté the onion, celery, carrots, and garlic for 5 minutes. Season with the salt and pepper.

2. Add the broth and chicken and cook for 10 minutes.

3. Turn off the heat. Remove the chicken and shred using two forks. Place the chicken back into the pot.

4. Add the diced tomatoes, tomato paste, and peas. Reduce heat to medium-low and cook for 5 minutes. Serve 1 cup of chicken stew over ½ cup of farro in individual bowls. Store leftovers in a sealed container in the refrigerator for up to 4 days.

Make it easier: If you have leftover chicken, this is a great dish to use it up with.

Per serving (1 cup stew + ½ cup farro): Calories: 425; Fat: 7.5g; Carbohydrates: 45g; Fiber: 7.5g; Sugar: 11g; Protein: 44g; Sodium: 1,020mg

Shrimp and Vegetable Wild Rice Bowl

Dairy-Free	Prep time: 10 minutes / Cook time: 45 minutes / Serves: 4

Wild rice is an excellent source of zinc, meeting 15 percent of your daily value per cooked cup. Zinc helps with the immune and digestive systems, helps control diabetes, reduces stress levels, and boosts metabolism. Enjoy its benefits in this flavorful bowl with shrimp and broccoli.

FOR THE WILD RICE

3 cups water

1 cup uncooked wild rice

½ teaspoon sea salt

FOR THE STIR-FRY

1 tablespoon canola oil

1 medium head broccoli, florets and stem chopped into bite-size pieces (about 3½ cups)

½ red onion, chopped

1 pound cooked shrimp, peeled and deveined

2 tablespoons reduced-sodium soy sauce

½ teaspoon sea salt

¼ teaspoon freshly ground black pepper

1 teaspoon sesame seeds

TO MAKE THE WILD RICE

1. In a large saucepan, bring the water to a boil.

2. Stir in the wild rice and salt. Reduce heat to a simmer and cook, covered, for 40 to 45 minutes, or just until the kernels puff open.

3. Uncover and fluff with a fork, then simmer for an additional 5 minutes. Remove from heat and drain any excess liquid. Keep covered until ready to use.

TO MAKE THE STIR-FRY

4. When the rice is about 15 minutes from being done, heat a large skillet over medium-high heat. In the skillet, heat the canola oil for 1 minute.

5. Add the broccoli and sauté for 5 minutes until broccoli is soft, stirring occasionally. Add the onion and cook, stirring occasionally, for an additional 2 minutes, until translucent.

6. Add the shrimp, soy sauce, salt, and pepper and cook for another 2 minutes, stirring frequently.

7. Divide the rice between 4 bowls, top with the stir-fry, and garnish with the sesame seeds before serving. Store leftovers in a sealed container in the refrigerator for up to 4 days.

Swap or substitute: You can use brown rice or quinoa instead of wild rice.

Per serving (1½ cups): **Calories:** 308; Fat: 4.5g; Carbohydrates: 34g; Fiber: 3.5g; Sugar: 2g; Protein: 35g; Sodium: 1,008mg

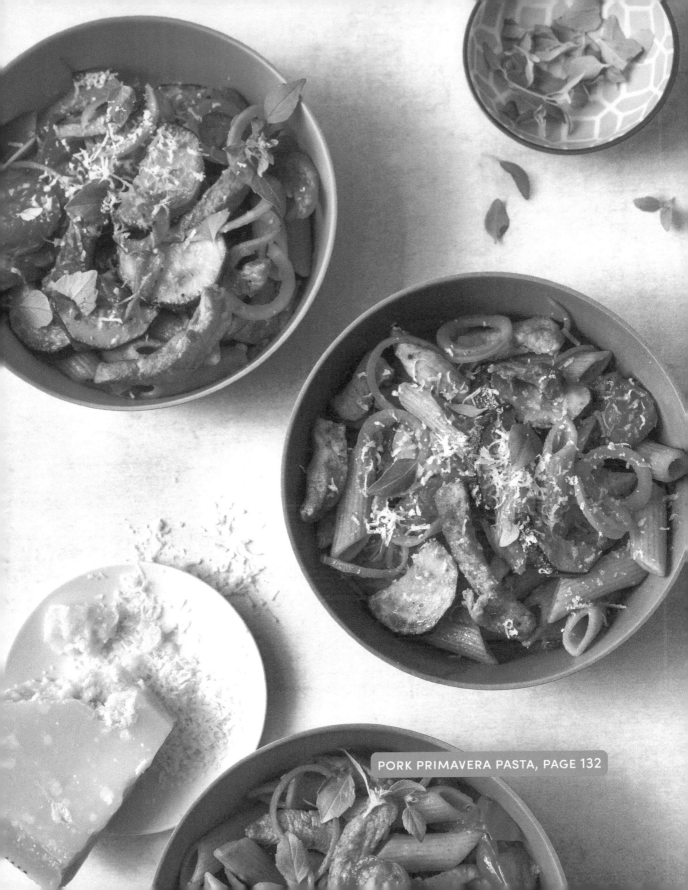

PORK PRIMAVERA PASTA, PAGE 132

CHAPTER SIX

DINNERS

Blackened Fish with Bean Salad 104

Sheet Pan Glazed Balsamic Salmon with Asparagus 105

Sheet Pan Roasted Tofu and Cauliflower 106

Sheet Pan Cracked-Egg Pizza 108

Sheet Pan Mediterranean Chicken with Butternut Squash 109

Fried Shrimp Brown Rice 110

Seafood à la Paella with Farro 111

Peruvian-Style Arroz con Pollo 113

Wild Fiesta Rice with Roasted Chicken 115

Mayo-Yogurt Baked Chicken with Mini Potatoes 116

Ground Turkey and Vegetable Stuffed Bell Peppers 118

Chickpea Stir-Fry 120

Beef and Vegetable Stir-Fry 121

Electric Pressure Cooker Chicken, White Beans,
Spinach, and Mushrooms in White Wine 122

Electric Pressure Cooker Low-Cal Beef Bourguignon 124

Electric Pressure Cooker Red Lentil Soup 126

Vegetable-Layered Cheese Lasagna 127

Lean Beef Meatballs in Tomato Sauce with Polenta 128

Glazed Pork Tenderloin and Bell Peppers 130

Pork Primavera Pasta 132

Blackened Fish with Bean Salad

Dairy-Free Gluten-Free	Prep time: 10 minutes / Cook time: 5 minutes / Serves: 4

You don't need a lot of fat and sugar to get bold flavors, and the spices in this recipe really shine. If you're looking for a restaurant-quality recipe without all the added fat and sugar, this is the meal for you.

FOR THE FISH

1 teaspoon garlic powder

1 teaspoon dried thyme

1 teaspoon dried oregano

1 teaspoon
   smoked paprika

½ teaspoon cumin

½ teaspoon freshly
   ground black pepper

½ teaspoon cayenne

1 pound tilapia fillets

1 tablespoon canola oil

FOR THE SALAD

1 cup frozen shelled
   edamame, thawed

1 cup frozen corn, thawed

1 cup frozen peas, thawed

2 (7-inch) carrots,
   thinly sliced

¼ cup diced red onion

⅔ cup Lemon-Mustard
   Vinaigrette (page 155)

TO MAKE THE FISH

1. In a medium bowl, combine the garlic powder, thyme, oregano, paprika, cumin, pepper, and cayenne and mix well.

2. Sprinkle all sides of the fish fillets with the seasoning mixture.

3. In a large skillet over medium heat, heat the oil. Fry the fish for 2 minutes on each side or until cooked through.

TO MAKE THE SALAD

4. In a large bowl, combine all the salad ingredients and mix well.

5. Serve the salad alongside the fish. Store leftovers in a sealed container in the refrigerator for up to 4 days.

> **Swap or substitute:** This recipe will apply to any whitefish, such as mahi-mahi or sole. Check to see what's on sale in your supermarket!

Per serving (3 ounces fish + 1 cup salad): Calories: 322; Fat: 14g; Carbohydrates: 22g; Fiber: 5.5g; Sugar: 5.5g; Protein: 30g; Sodium: 392mg

Sheet Pan Glazed Balsamic Salmon with Asparagus

Dairy-Free Gluten-Free	Prep time: 10 minutes / Cook time: 15 minutes / Serves: 4

Sheet pan recipes are a great way to cook your favorite protein with a vegetable at the same time, with minimal cleanup required. You'll want to pick a vegetable that will cook at the same speed as the protein so they both cook evenly. For example, cooking potatoes with fish would not be ideal, because the fish will cook faster.

Nonstick cooking spray

1 pound boneless, skinless salmon fillets

¾ teaspoon sea salt, divided

¼ teaspoon freshly ground black pepper

¼ teaspoon garlic powder

1 tablespoon balsamic vinegar glaze

16 asparagus spears

1. Preheat the oven to 450°F. Cover a large baking sheet with aluminum foil and spray it with cooking spray.

2. On one side of the baking sheet, sprinkle the salmon with ½ teaspoon of salt, pepper, and garlic powder. Using your hands, smear the balsamic glaze over the salmon, making sure to cover the top of the fish.

3. On the other side of the baking sheet, sprinkle the asparagus with the remaining ¼ teaspoon of salt.

4. Bake for 12 minutes, or until the fish flakes when pressed with a fork. Serve the salmon with the asparagus on the side. Store leftovers in a sealed container in the refrigerator for up to 4 days.

Per serving (3 ounces salmon + 4 asparagus):
Calories: 230; Fat: 12g; Carbohydrates: 4g; Fiber: 1.5g;
Sugar: 2g; Protein: 27g; Sodium: 494mg

Sheet Pan Roasted Tofu and Cauliflower

Dairy-Free Vegan	**Prep time:** 10 minutes, plus 30 minutes to marinate / **Cook time:** 55 minutes / **Serves:** 3

Here's a delicious and satisfying vegan option for meatless Mondays. Cook the tofu on a weekend and use it throughout the week to add to salads, grain dishes, vegetable dishes, or any dish where you want some plant-based protein.

2 garlic cloves, crushed

2 tablespoons white vinegar

1 tablespoon reduced-sodium soy sauce

1 (14-ounce) block extra-firm tofu, drained

Nonstick cooking spray

1 head cauliflower, cut into florets

½ teaspoon garlic powder

½ teaspoon sea salt

¼ teaspoon freshly ground black pepper

1. Preheat the oven to 450°F.

2. In a large, shallow bowl, combine the garlic, vinegar, and soy sauce. Mix with a fork until smooth. Set aside.

3. Slice the drained tofu into six ½-inch slabs. Dip each piece of tofu in the marinade, making sure to coat all sides completely. Let the tofu rest in the marinade for 30 minutes. (The tofu can also marinate overnight in the refrigerator.)

4. Line a large baking sheet with aluminum foil and spray the foil with cooking spray. On one side of the sheet pan, place the pieces of tofu ½-inch apart. Pour the remaining marinade over each piece of tofu.

5. On the other side of the baking sheet, arrange the cauliflower in a single layer and sprinkle it with the garlic powder, salt, and pepper. Spray with nonstick cooking spray.

6. Roast for 25 minutes or until the tofu is crisp and golden around the edges. Let cool slightly before serving.

Store it: Roasted tofu can be stored in a sealed container in the refrigerator for up to 4 days. Enjoy it hot or cold.

Per serving (2 slices tofu + 1 cup cauliflower): Calories: 185; Fat: 7.5g; Carbohydrates: 14g; Fiber: 5.5g; Sugar: 5.5g; Protein: 18g; Sodium: 644mg

Sheet Pan Cracked-Egg Pizza

Vegetarian	Prep time: 10 minutes / Cook time: 20 minutes / Serves: 2

Flatbreads are also called "lavash bread." You can find many brands in the grocery store, but look for flatbreads that are 120 calories or fewer per sheet and with at least 3 grams of fiber. They serve as the base for these colorful and inventive pizzas.

Nonstick cooking spray

2 whole-grain flatbreads or lavash bread

¼ cup canned pizza sauce

¼ cup canned diced tomatoes

2 tablespoons dried oregano

3 ounces shredded part-skim mozzarella cheese

¼ red onion, sliced

½ yellow bell pepper, sliced

½ red bell pepper, sliced

4 large eggs

½ cup arugula

1. Preheat the oven to 400°F. Spray a baking sheet with cooking spray and place the flatbreads on top.

2. Spread half the pizza sauce and diced tomatoes on each of the flatbreads. Sprinkle with oregano to taste. Evenly distribute the cheese, onion, and yellow and red bell peppers across the flatbreads.

3. On each flatbread, move the vegetables to clear out two "beds" to place the eggs. Crack an egg into each of the "beds," 2 eggs per flatbread.

4. Bake for about 15 minutes, or until golden brown and the eggs are set. Remove from the oven, top with the arugula, and let cool for 5 minutes before enjoying.

Store it: Store leftovers in a sealed container in the refrigerator for breakfast the next day. These pizzas will keep for up to 2 days.

Per serving (1 flatbread pizza): Calories: 480; Fat: 28g; Carbohydrates: 31g; Fiber: 11g; Sugar: 7.5g; Protein: 34g; Sodium: 852mg

Sheet Pan Mediterranean Chicken with Butternut Squash

Dairy-Free Gluten-Free	Prep time: 15 minutes / Cook time: 15 minutes / Serves: 4

Sheet pan recipes are a theme in this book because they are one of my favorite ways to cook. A big plus of making your meals on a sheet pan is the easy cleanup, giving you more time to get your workouts in. And if you haven't tried roasted butternut squash, you're in for a treat. See page 148 for instructions on how to butterfly chicken.

Nonstick cooking spray

1 pound boneless, skinless chicken breasts, butterflied

1 tablespoon dried oregano

1 teaspoon lemon juice

1 teaspoon extra-virgin olive oil

½ teaspoon sea salt, divided

¼ teaspoon freshly ground black pepper, plus more for seasoning

¼ teaspoon garlic powder

1 pound butternut squash, peeled, seeded, and cut into 1-inch cubes

1. Preheat the oven to 450°F. Line a large baking sheet with aluminum foil and spray the foil with nonstick cooking spray. Set aside.

2. In a small bowl, stir together the chicken, oregano, lemon juice, olive oil, ¼ teaspoon of salt, pepper, and garlic powder, coating the chicken well.

3. On one side of the baking sheet, place the chicken in a single layer. On the other side of the baking sheet, arrange the butternut squash in a single layer, sprinkle the squash with the remaining ¼ teaspoon of salt, and season with pepper to taste. Spray the chicken and squash with nonstick spray.

4. Bake for 14 minutes, or until juices run clear and squash is soft. Serve the chicken with the squash on the side.

Store it: Store leftovers in a sealed container in the refrigerator for up to 4 days, or in the freezer for up to 3 months.

Per serving (3 ounces chicken + ½ cup squash): Calories: 225; Fat: 11g; Carbohydrates: 11g; Fiber: 2g; Sugar: 2g; Protein: 24g; Sodium: 349mg

Fried Shrimp Brown Rice

Dairy-Free	Prep time: 10 minutes / Cook time: 20 minutes / Serves: 4

Arroz chaufa is fried rice, born from the Chinese influence on Peruvian cuisine. Peru's cuisine was also influenced by French, Spanish, and Italian cultures. I grew up eating fried rice, and I still love flavors from around the world and use them in this book.

3 large eggs

⅛ teaspoon sea salt

Nonstick cooking spray

1 tablespoon sesame oil

2 (12-inch) celery stalks, diced

1 cup shredded carrots

¼ cup diced red onion

1 teaspoon crushed ginger

½ teaspoon minced garlic

2 tablespoons reduced-sodium soy sauce

¼ teaspoon sea salt

1 pound large (20 to 25 count) shrimp, peeled and deveined

1 cup frozen peas

4 scallions, green and white parts, diced

2 cups Basic Brown Rice (page 150)

1. In a small bowl, whisk together the eggs and salt.

2. Heat a large skillet over medium heat and spray lightly with cooking spray. Pour the eggs into the skillet and cook for about 5 minutes, making a rough omelet. Set the skillet aside to cool for 5 minutes and chop the omelet into 1-inch pieces.

3. In the skillet, heat the sesame oil over medium heat. Add the celery, carrots, red onion, ginger, and garlic and sauté, stirring occasionally, for 5 minutes or until soft. Stir in the soy sauce and salt.

4. Add the shrimp and peas, increase heat to high, and cook for 3 minutes, turning the shrimp to cook on both sides.

5. Stir in the scallions, eggs, and rice and mix well. Cook for another 2 minutes. Serve.

Store it: Store leftovers in a sealed container in the refrigerator for up to 4 days.

Per serving (1½ cups): Calories: 342; Fat: 10g; Carbohydrates: 36g; Fiber: 4.5g; Sugar: 5g; Protein: 28g; Sodium: 897mg

Seafood à la Paella with Farro

Dairy-Free	Prep time: 10 minutes / Cook time: 10 minutes / Serves: 6

When I visited Barcelona, I fell in love with the flavors of seafood paella. I wanted to create a way to fit those delicious paella flavors into low-calorie eating, and thus this extraordinary recipe was born.

1 tablespoon extra-virgin olive oil, divided

8 ounces sole fillet

4 ounces scallops, any type

1 large white onion, diced

1 medium red bell pepper, diced

1 (14½-ounce) can diced tomatoes, drained

1 cup frozen peas, thawed

1½ teaspoons sea salt

1 teaspoon smoked paprika

¼ teaspoon saffron

¼ teaspoon freshly ground black pepper

1 pound large (20 to 25 count) shrimp, peeled and deveined

3 cups Basic Farro (page 149)

1. In a large, deep skillet over medium-high heat, heat ½ tablespoon of oil and panfry the sole and scallops for 1 minute on each side. Remove the fish and scallops and set them aside.

2. In the skillet, heat the remaining ½ tablespoon of oil. Add the onion and bell peppers and cook, stirring occasionally, for about 5 minutes.

3. Add the tomatoes, peas, salt, paprika, saffron, and pepper and mix well.

4. Add the shrimp and mix well. Cook for 2 minutes.

5. Add the farro and mix well. Place the fish and scallops on top and mix gently. Cover and simmer on low heat for 2 minutes, then serve. Store leftovers in a sealed container in the refrigerator for up to 4 days.

Per serving (1½ cups): Calories: 281; Fat: 4.5g; Carbohydrates: 33g; Fiber: 4.5g; Sugar: 5g; Protein: 27g; Sodium: 1,234mg

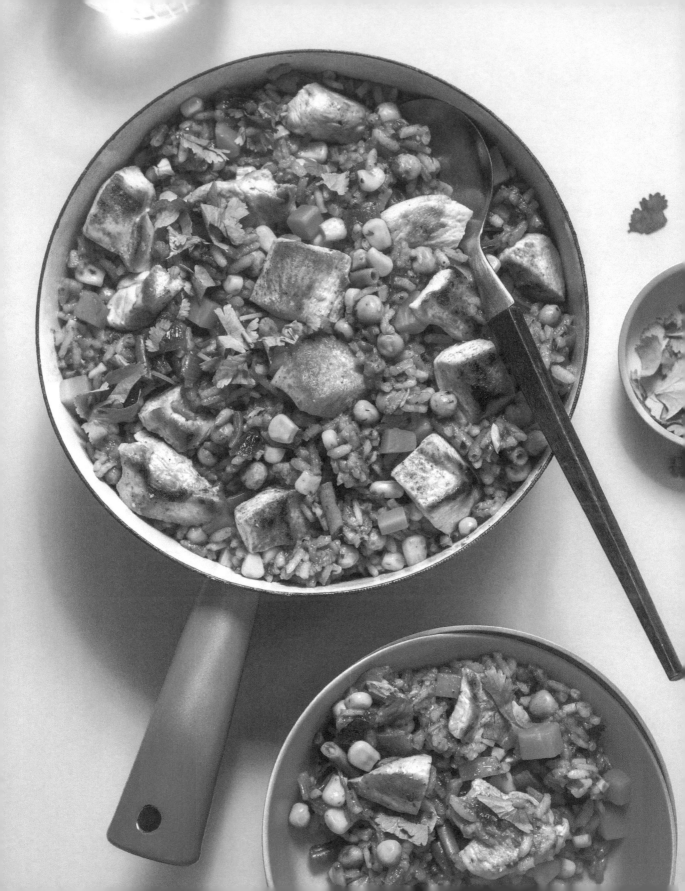

Peruvian-Style Arroz con Pollo

Dairy-Free	**Prep time:** 20 minutes / **Cook time:** 35 minutes / **Serves:** 4

This is one of the first dishes I learned how to cook, so as you can imagine, it brings me warm memories of my home in Peru. Even though you could call this my "comfort food," it's low in calories but big in flavor. I recommend using mixed frozen corn, green beans, and carrots. Garnish with more fresh cilantro before serving, if desired.

1 tablespoon canola oil, divided

1 pound boneless, skinless chicken breast, cut into bite-size cubes

1 medium red onion, diced

2 cups cilantro leaves

1 cup chicken broth

1 teaspoon garlic, minced

1 tablespoon aji amarillo chili paste or other chili paste

1½ teaspoons sea salt

½ teaspoon cumin

½ teaspoon freshly ground black pepper

1 cup long-grain white rice

1 cup dark beer

3 cups frozen mixed vegetables

1 medium bell pepper, any color, thinly sliced

1. Heat a large, deep skillet over medium-high heat. In the skillet, heat ½ tablespoon of canola oil for 1 minute. Add the chicken and cook for about 2 minutes on each side, or until it begins to get a good sear. Remove the chicken and set aside.

2. Add the remaining ½ tablespoon of canola oil and the onion. Reduce heat to medium-low and cook, stirring occasionally, for 4 minutes, until the onion is translucent.

3. While the onion cooks, put the cilantro and chicken broth in a blender and purée until the cilantro is well blended. Set aside.

4. Add the garlic, chili paste, salt, cumin, and pepper to the skillet with the onion and cook for 1 minute. Add the rice and stir, then add the cilantro mixture, beer, mixed vegetables, and bell pepper. Stir, bring to a boil, and reduce heat to low-medium.

CONTINUED

5. Add the chicken breast back on top of the rice, submerging it a bit. Cook for 25 to 30 minutes or until the rice is cooked. Mix well and serve.

Store it: This is a great meal for leftovers as it holds up very well. Consider making this recipe on the weekend and using it for meal prep throughout the week. Store leftovers in a sealed container in the refrigerator for up to 4 days.

Per serving (2 cups): **Calories: 456**; Fat: 7.5g; Carbohydrates: 60g; Fiber: 4.5g; Sugar: 7.5g; Protein: 33g; Sodium: 1,241mg

Wild Fiesta Rice with Roasted Chicken

Dairy-Free Gluten-Free	Prep time: 5 minutes / Cook time: 10 minutes / Serves: 4

If you enjoy dishes with a multitude of textures and flavors, get ready for a treat. The wild rice in this recipe adds a beautiful color to the dish when combined with the vegetables and is also rich in fiber. Fiber is beneficial for heart and gut health and slows digestion, helping you feel fuller for longer.

1 tablespoon extra-virgin olive oil

1 cup diced red bell pepper

1 medium white onion, chopped

1 teaspoon sea salt

½ cup chopped walnuts

½ cup golden raisins

¼ cup finely diced parsley

2 cups cooked wild rice (page 100)

12 ounces Roasted Chicken (page 148) or rotisserie chicken

1. In a large skillet over medium heat, heat the oil. Add the bell pepper, onion, and salt and cook, stirring occasionally, for 5 minutes, until the onion is translucent.

2. Add the walnuts and raisins. Cook, stirring occasionally, until lightly browned and fragrant, about 2 minutes.

3. In a large bowl, combine the sautéed mixture, parsley, and wild rice. Stir to combine. Serve topped with the roasted chicken.

Store it: Store leftovers in a sealed container in the refrigerator for up to 4 days.

Per serving (1¼ cups rice + 3 ounces chicken):
Calories: 428; Fat: 17g; Carbohydrates: 41g; Fiber: 4.5g; Sugar: 16g; Protein: 30g; Sodium: 1,228mg

Mayo-Yogurt Baked Chicken with Mini Potatoes

Gluten-Free	**Prep time:** 15 minutes, plus 20 minutes to marinate / **Cook time:** 35 minutes / **Serves:** 4

We Peruvians love our potatoes, so of course I had to include potato salad in this book. This recipe features purple potatoes, which have more anti-oxidants than your traditional potatoes and are native to Peru.

¼ cup plain 2% Greek yogurt

¼ cup avocado oil mayonnaise

1 teaspoon sea salt, divided

½ teaspoon freshly ground black pepper, divided

1 pound boneless, skinless chicken breast, butterflied (see page 148 for instructions on how to butterfly chicken)

20 ounces purple mini potatoes, thinly sliced

¼ teaspoon garlic powder

Nonstick cooking spray

1. Preheat the oven to 450°F.

2. In a large bowl, stir together the yogurt, mayonnaise, ½ teaspoon of salt, and ¼ teaspoon of pepper until well blended.

3. Add the chicken, stirring to make sure the poultry is completely coated. Cover with plastic wrap and let sit for 20 minutes.

4. In a medium bowl, combine the potatoes and the remaining ½ teaspoon of salt, ¼ teaspoon pepper, and the garlic powder. Mix well to coat all the potatoes.

5. Spray a large roasting pan with nonstick cooking spray. Transfer the chicken breasts and potatoes into the roasting pan, spreading them in a single layer.

6. Bake for 15 minutes or until the chicken is done with no pink remaining. Serve warm. Store leftovers in a sealed container in the refrigerator for up to 4 days.

Swap or substitute: By using Greek yogurt instead of all mayonnaise like a traditional potato salad recipe would use, you cut down on the calories and fat, while also getting a boost of lean protein.

Per serving (3 ounces chicken + ¾ cup potatoes): Calories: 327; Fat: 15g; Carbohydrates: 23g; Fiber: 3.5g; Sugar: 2.5g; Protein: 26g; Sodium: 766mg

Ground Turkey and Vegetable Stuffed Bell Peppers

Dairy-Free **Gluten-Free**	**Prep time:** 15 minutes / **Cook time:** 40 minutes / **Serves:** 4

If there's a dish everyone seems to love, it's stuffed bell peppers. The combination of turkey, veggies, and more veggies in this dish means you won't have to worry about hitting your daily vegetable servings with this dinner on the menu! Consider using a variety of colored peppers for even more visual appeal.

1 tablespoon extra-virgin olive oil

½ cup chopped red onion

1 teaspoon crushed ginger

1 teaspoon crushed garlic

2 (6-inch) celery stalks, diced

1 (6-inch) zucchini, diced

1 pound ground turkey

¼ teaspoon sea salt

⅛ teaspoon freshly ground black pepper

1 (14½-ounce) can diced tomatoes

1 cup frozen peas

4 large bell peppers, any color, tops cut off

1. Preheat the oven to 400°F. Line a 9-inch-by-13-inch baking dish with aluminum foil and set aside.

2. In a large skillet over medium heat, heat the oil. Add the onion, ginger, and garlic and cook for 2 minutes, stirring occasionally, until the onion is translucent.

3. Add the celery and zucchini and sauté for 3 minutes, stirring occasionally, until the vegetables are soft.

4. Stir in the ground turkey and sauté, breaking apart with a spoon, until cooked through, about 6 minutes. Season the mixture with salt and pepper. Add the tomatoes and peas and mix well.

5. Evenly divide the ground turkey mixture between the bell peppers. In the baking dish, arrange the stuffed bell peppers upright and cover them with aluminum foil. Bake for 20 minutes.

6. Remove the dish from the oven and carefully remove the aluminum foil. Place back in the oven and cook for another 10 minutes or until the peppers are tender. Serve warm.

Store it: Store leftovers in a sealed container in the refrigerator for up to 4 days.

Per serving (1 stuffed pepper): **Calories:** 302; Fat: 13g; Carbohydrates: 21g; Fiber: 6.5g; Sugar: 11g; Protein: 27g; Sodium: 493mg

Chickpea Stir-Fry

Dairy-Free **Vegan**	**Prep time:** 10 minutes / **Cook time:** 10 minutes / **Serves:** 4

We've all had chicken stir-fry, but have you ever tried a chickpea stir-fry? Another idea for your meatless Mondays, this stir-fry also delivers a dose of good fiber and all the wonderful antioxidants you find in legumes. Chickpeas also go by the name garbanzo beans.

1 tablespoon canola oil

1 large red onion, cut into strips

3 bell peppers, any color, cut into strips

3 (15-ounce) cans chickpeas, drained

1 teaspoon cumin

1 teaspoon ground turmeric

1 teaspoon freshly ground black pepper

½ teaspoon garlic powder

3 tablespoons reduced-sodium soy sauce

1 tablespoon balsamic vinegar

2 tomatoes, cut into strips

½ cup chopped cilantro

1. Heat a large skillet over high heat for 1 minute. Put the oil, onion, and bell peppers in the skillet and cook for 4 minutes, stirring frequently.

2. Add the chickpeas and stir. Cook for an additional minute.

3. Add the cumin, turmeric, pepper, and garlic powder. Stir well to incorporate all the spices.

4. Add the soy sauce and vinegar. Cook, stirring frequently, for 2 minutes.

5. Add the tomato and cilantro and cook for 1 minute longer. Serve.

Store it: Store leftovers in a sealed container in the refrigerator for up to 4 days.

Per serving (2 cups): Calories: 361; Fat: 9g; Carbohydrates: 57g; Fiber: 16g; Sugar: 14g; Protein: 17g; Sodium: 864mg

Beef and Vegetable Stir-Fry

Dairy-Free	**Prep time:** 10 minutes / **Cook time:** 10 minutes / **Serves:** 6

Lomo saltado is a popular beef stir-fry dish served in restaurants and homes throughout Peru. Part of a fusion of Chinese and Peruvian cultures known as *chifa*, this stir-fry combines sliced steak with soy sauce, herbs, and vegetables cut into sticks.

1 tablespoon canola oil

2 pounds top sirloin or filet mignon, thinly sliced into stick-shaped pieces

1 teaspoon cumin

1 teaspoon sea salt

¼ teaspoon freshly ground black pepper

1 red onion, cut into sticks

1 teaspoon crushed garlic

2 tablespoons balsamic vinegar

1 tablespoon aji amarillo chili paste (or any chili paste)

3 Roma tomatoes, cut into sticks

3 tablespoons reduced-sodium soy sauce

½ cup cilantro leaves

1. In a large skillet over high heat, heat the oil and sauté the beef for 3 minutes until browned, turning to cook all sides. Add the cumin, salt, and pepper and mix well. Remove the meat and set aside.

2. In the same skillet, combine the onion, garlic, vinegar, and chili paste. Cook for 5 minutes, stirring well. Add the tomatoes and mix well.

3. Return the beef to the pan, add the soy sauce, mix well, and cook for another minute. Sprinkle with cilantro before serving. Store leftovers in a sealed container in the refrigerator for up to 4 days.

Bulk it up: If you'd like to add a carbohydrate, ½ cup to 1 cup of a grain such as brown rice or quinoa makes an excellent addition. Just make sure it fits into your calories for the day.

Per serving (1⅓ cups): Calories: 238; Fat: 8.5g; Carbohydrates: 4g; Fiber: 0.5g; Sugar: 2.5g; Protein: 36g; Sodium: 821mg

Electric Pressure Cooker Chicken, White Beans, Spinach, and Mushrooms in White Wine

Dairy-Free	Prep time: 10 minutes / Cook time: 15 minutes / Serves: 6

Let's face it—a lot of international dishes are simply not weight loss friendly. However, this French-inspired chicken dish is not one of those. The use of the electric pressure cooker allows all of those French flavors to develop in only a fraction of the time. See the tip for stovetop directions.

1 tablespoon extra-virgin olive oil

4 (6-inch) carrots, sliced

10 ounces sliced mushrooms

1 medium red onion, chopped

1 teaspoon chopped garlic

1 cup white cooking wine

¼ cup chicken broth

¼ cup lemon juice

2 tablespoons cornstarch

2 pounds boneless, skinless chicken breast, cubed (2-inch)

1. Select the sauté option on the pressure cooker. In the pressure cooker, sauté the oil, carrots, mushrooms, onion, and garlic for 5 minutes, stirring occasionally.

2. Pour in the wine, broth, and lemon juice and mix well. Using a sieve, sift in the cornstarch and mix well.

3. Add the chicken, basil, salt, and pepper and mix well.

4. Close and cook on "manual" high pressure for 5 minutes. When done, turn the pressure valve to release the steam and open the lid.

1 cup packed whole
basil leaves

2 teaspoons sea salt

½ teaspoon freshly ground
black pepper

2 (15½-ounce) cans white
beans, drained and rinsed

6 cups spinach

5. Add the beans and spinach and mix well. Cook on "manual" high pressure for 2 minutes. When done, turn the pressure valve to release the steam and open the lid. Serve. Store leftovers in a sealed container in the refrigerator for up to 4 days.

Swap or substitute: This soup can also be made on the stovetop. Cook as directed, but increase the cook time in step 3 to 20 to 25 minutes.

Per serving (1½ cups): **Calories:** 411; **Fat:** 6.5g; **Carbohydrates:** 35g; **Fiber:** 10g; **Sugar:** 6g; **Protein:** 46g; **Sodium:** 1,584mg

Electric Pressure Cooker Low-Cal Beef Bourguignon

Dairy-Free	**Prep time:** 15 minutes / **Cook time:** 50 minutes / **Serves:** 6

Although I've also included stovetop directions (see tip), an electric pressure cooker makes quick work of this typically time-consuming classic dish, and it still has all of those stunning French flavors. A bouquet garni is a bundle of herbs added to casseroles, stocks, sauces, and soups. For ours, we'll use parsley, basil, and celery sticks.

1 tablespoon extra-virgin olive oil, divided

1 large white onion, chopped

4 (6-inch) carrots, sliced

1 teaspoon crushed garlic

4 tablespoons cornstarch, divided

1½ cups red wine

1 cup beef broth

1 (6-ounce) can tomato paste

2 pounds lean stew beef

1 small bunch parsley

1 small bunch basil

2 (12-inch) celery stalks, cut in half

8 ounces sliced mushrooms

10 ounces pearl onions

2 teaspoons sea salt

½ teaspoon freshly ground black pepper

1. Select the "sauté" function on the pressure cooker and add ½ tablespoon of oil, the onion, the carrots, and the garlic. Sauté for 4 minutes, stirring occasionally.

2. Using a sieve, sift in 2 tablespoons of cornstarch and mix well with the sauté mixture.

3. Pour in the wine, broth, and tomato paste and mix well. Add the beef and mix well. Gather the parsley, basil, and celery in a bunch, place it in the cooker, and submerge it a bit.

4. Close and cook on "manual" high pressure for 40 minutes. When done, turn the pressure valve to release the steam and open the lid.

5. In a large skillet over medium heat, heat the remaining ½ tablespoon of oil. In the skillet, sauté the mushrooms and pearl onions, stirring occasionally, for about 5 minutes or until brown.

6. Add the pearl onions and mushrooms to the electric pressure cooker and mix well. Cook on "manual" high pressure for 5 minutes. When done, turn the pressure valve to release the steam and open the lid.

7. Remove the garni and, using a sieve, sift in the remaining 2 tablespoons of cornstarch. Mix well before serving. Store leftovers in a sealed container in the refrigerator for up to 4 days, or freeze for up to 3 months.

Swap or substitute: To cook this on the stovetop, follow the same steps but increase the beef broth to 4 cups and simmer the stew over low heat, covered, for 3 hours.

Per serving (1⅓ cups): **Calories: 374**; Fat: 10g; Carbohydrates: 26g; Fiber: 4.5g; Sugar: 9.5g; Protein: 36g; Sodium: 1,245mg

Electric Pressure Cooker Red Lentil Soup

Dairy-Free Gluten-Free Vegan	Prep time: 10 minutes Cook time: 10 minutes Serves: 6

Inspired by a traditional Indian dish, this soup is one of my go-to dinners on those cooler nights or even as a warm lunch on chilly, stay-at-home afternoons. Feel free to use chicken broth in place of the vegetable if you prefer. See the tip for stovetop directions.

1 tablespoon extra-virgin olive oil

1 medium red onion, diced

4 (12-inch) celery stalks, sliced

3 (6-inch) carrots, sliced

1 (14½-ounce) can diced tomatoes

2 cups dry red lentils

1 cup frozen corn

2 teaspoons sea salt

1 teaspoon crushed garlic

1 teaspoon crushed ginger

1 teaspoon cumin

1 teaspoon turmeric powder

½ teaspoon freshly ground black pepper

4 cups vegetable broth

6 cups spinach

½ cup chopped cilantro

1. Select the sauté option on the pressure cooker. In the pressure cooker, sauté the onion in the oil, stirring occasionally, for 4 minutes, or until the onion is translucent.

2. Add the celery, carrots, tomatoes, lentils, corn, salt, garlic, ginger, cumin, turmeric, and pepper, then add the broth.

3. Close and cook on "manual" high pressure for 5 minutes. When done, turn the pressure valve to release the steam and open the lid.

4. Add the spinach and cilantro and mix well until the spinach is wilted. Serve. Store leftovers in a sealed container in the refrigerator for up to 4 days.

Swap or substitute: This soup can also be made on the stovetop. Cook as directed, but increase the cook time in step 3 to 20 to 25 minutes.

Per serving (2 cups): Calories: **328**; Fat: 4g; Carbohydrates: 57g; Fiber: 11g; Sugar: 6g; Protein: 18g; Sodium: 1,372mg

Vegetable-Layered Cheese Lasagna

Vegetarian Gluten-Free	Prep time: 15 minutes / Cook time: 45 minutes / Serves: 6

Zucchini noodles are a fantastic and clever way to add more veggies to your day. Even though this Italian dish is absent of pasta, it's not missing any of those delicious Italian flavors. Your entire family will love this lasagna.

3 cups part-skim ricotta cheese

½ teaspoon sea salt

¼ teaspoon freshly ground black pepper

1½ tablespoons cornstarch

¼ cup warm water

Nonstick cooking spray

1 medium eggplant, cut into ¼-inch slices

2 cups sliced baby bella mushrooms

2 cups spinach

3 (8-inch) zucchini, cut into ¼-inch slices

1 (14½-ounce) can diced, no-salt-added tomatoes, drained

1 cup basil leaves

1 tablespoon dried oregano

1 cup shredded part-skim mozzarella cheese

1 cup shredded Parmesan cheese

1. Preheat the oven to 450°F.

2. In a medium bowl, stir together the ricotta, salt, pepper, cornstarch, and water. Set aside.

3. Spray a 9-by-13-inch baking dish with nonstick spray. In the prepared baking dish, place the eggplant slices in the dish, followed by the ricotta mixture. Lay the mushrooms and spinach on top of the ricotta mixture.

4. Next, layer half of the zucchini slices followed by the tomatoes, basil, and oregano. Sprinkle the mozzarella on top.

5. Lay the other half of the zucchini slices and sprinkle the Parmesan cheese on top. Cover the dish with aluminum foil and bake for 30 minutes.

6. Remove the aluminum foil and bake for another 15 minutes before serving. Cut the lasagna into six 4-inch squares.

Store it: Store leftovers in a sealed container in the refrigerator for up to 4 days. It can also be frozen for up to 3 months.

Per serving (1 square): **Calories: 394**; Fat: 21g; Carbohydrates: 29g; Fiber: 7g; Sugar: 10g; Protein: 28g; Sodium: 718mg

Lean Beef Meatballs in Tomato Sauce with Polenta

Gluten-Free	Prep time: 15 minutes / Cook time: 40 minutes / Serves: 4

Polenta is a type of degerminated cornmeal popular in Italian cuisine. This recipe makes a tasty and filling meal, but you can always just cook the polenta and have it with other foods, such as fried eggs.

4 cups water

2 teaspoons sea salt, divided

1 cup dry polenta

1 pound 93% lean ground beef

5 ounces sliced baby bella mushrooms

½ cup 1% milk

½ cup shredded Parmesan cheese

1 tablespoon dried oregano

1 teaspoon minced garlic

½ teaspoon freshly ground black pepper

1 (14½-ounce) can diced tomatoes

½ (6-ounce) can tomato paste

1. In a 4-quart saucepan, bring the water to a boil with 1 teaspoon of sea salt. Gradually add the polenta to the boiling water, stirring frequently until thickened, about 25 minutes.

2. Meanwhile, in a large bowl, combine the beef, mushrooms, milk, Parmesan, oregano, garlic, the remaining teaspoon of salt, and the pepper. Use your hands to mix, making sure all the ingredients are well distributed.

3. Scoop the meat mixture using a ¼-cup measuring cup and use wet hands to roll it into 2-inch meatballs.

4. In a 4-quart pot over medium heat, combine the tomatoes and tomato paste and stir well. Add the meatballs to the sauce and cook for 30 minutes.

5. Serve the meatballs and sauce over the polenta. Store leftovers in a sealed container in the refrigerator for up to 4 days.

Swap or substitute: If you can't find polenta in your supermarket, you can substitute farro or brown rice.

Per serving (2 meatballs + 1 cup polenta + ⅓ cup sauce): Calories: 408; Fat: 12g; Carbohydrates: 41g; Fiber: 4g; Sugar: 8g; Protein: 33g; Sodium: 1,730mg

Glazed Pork Tenderloin and Bell Peppers

Dairy-Free Gluten-Free	Prep time: 10 minutes, plus 20 minutes to marinate / Cook time: 15 minutes / Serves: 5

If you're bored with endless chicken breasts in your weight loss plan, pork loin is a great source of lean protein with even less saturated fat than chicken breast. This quick, one-pan meal allows you to whip up a delicious, low-calorie pork dinner in no time.

1 tablespoon extra-virgin olive oil, divided

4 tablespoons balsamic vinegar glaze, divided

1 teaspoon crushed garlic

1 tablespoon crushed ginger

1 teaspoon sea salt, divided

¼ teaspoon freshly ground black pepper

1½ pounds pork tenderloin, trimmed and cut crosswise into 1-inch-thick slices

1 medium red bell pepper, cut into thin strips

1 medium yellow bell pepper, cut into thin strips

1 medium yellow onion, thinly sliced

1. In a small bowl, combine ½ tablespoon of oil, 2 tablespoons of balsamic glaze, the garlic, ginger, ½ teaspoon of salt, and the pepper, and mix well.

2. In a zip-top plastic bag, pour in the marinade mixture over the pork slices. Massage to combine well, making sure all the pork is covered with the mixture. Marinate for about 20 minutes.

3. In a large skillet over medium heat, heat the remaining ½ tablespoon of oil. Add the vegetables, the remaining 2 tablespoons of balsamic vinegar glaze, and the remaining ½ teaspoon of salt. Sauté, stirring occasionally, for about 7 minutes or until they are soft. Transfer to a serving dish and cover with aluminum foil until ready to serve.

4. Using the same skillet, cook the pork over medium-low heat for 6 minutes on each side or until it is no longer pink.

5. Serve the pork alongside the vegetables. Store leftovers in a sealed container in the refrigerator for up to 4 days.

Bulk it up: If you'd like to add a carbohydrate source to this meal, ½ cup to 1 cup of brown rice or quinoa makes an excellent addition. Just make sure it fits into your calories for the day.

Per serving (4 ounces pork + ¾ cup vegetables): Calories: 220; Fat: 7g; Carbohydrates: 9g; Fiber: 1g; Sugar: 5g; Protein: 28g; Sodium: 527mg

Pork Primavera Pasta

Prep time: 10 minutes, plus 20 minutes to marinate /
Cook time: 15 minutes / **Serves:** 6

Pasta lovers, get ready for a treat! I recommend using pasta with higher protein. Usually these kinds of pasta are made with chickpea or quinoa flour in addition to semolina and provide about 10 grams of protein per serving, more than traditional pasta.

8 ounces whole-grain protein-enriched penne pasta

¼ cup white cooking wine

2 tablespoons yellow mustard

½ teaspoon sea salt

½ teaspoon garlic powder

¼ cup freshly ground black pepper

1 pound boneless top loin pork chop, thinly cut into strips

1 tablespoon extra-virgin olive oil

¼ diced red onion

1 teaspoon chopped garlic

2 (7-inch) zucchini, cut into ½-inch slices

1 cup shredded carrots

1 teaspoon sea salt

2 cups cherry tomatoes, halved

½ cup chopped fresh basil

½ cup shredded Parmesan cheese

1. Bring a large pot of water to a boil. Cook the pasta according to package instructions for al dente. Drain and set aside.

2. While the pasta is cooking, in a large bowl, mix together the wine, mustard, salt, garlic powder, and pepper. Add the pork, stirring to coat, and let it marinate for at least 20 minutes.

3. Discard the marinade and, in a large skillet over medium heat, heat the oil. In the skillet, fry the pork for about 3 minutes, turning to cook on all sides. Set aside.

4. In the same skillet, cook the onion and garlic, stirring occasionally, for another 3 minutes, or until onion is translucent. Add the zucchini, carrots, and salt and sauté, stirring occasionally, for 10 minutes, or until the vegetables are softened.

5. Stir in the cherry tomatoes and basil and cook for another minute. Add the pork and mix well.

6. Add the pasta to the pork and vegetable mixture and toss to combine. Top with Parmesan before serving.

Store it: Store leftovers in a sealed container in the refrigerator for up to 4 days.

Per serving (1½ cups): **Calories:** 329; Fat: 11g; Carbohydrates: 33g; Fiber: 1.5g; Sugar: 4.5g; Protein: 26g; Sodium: 638mg

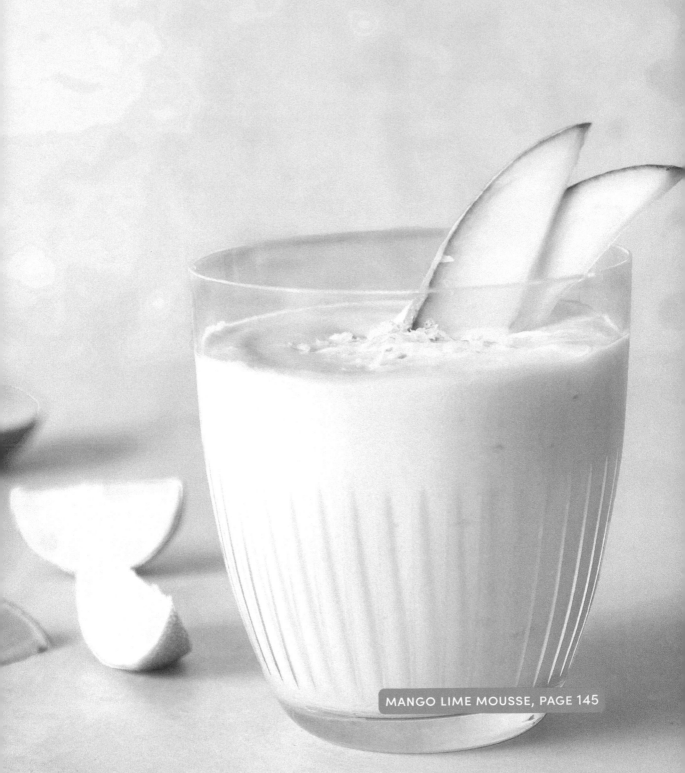

MANGO LIME MOUSSE, PAGE 145

CHAPTER SEVEN

SNACKS AND DESSERTS

Mixed Dried Fruit with Parmesan Cheese 136

Mini Parfait 137

Applesauce with Seeds 138

Hard-Boiled Egg and Apple Slices 139

Mason Jar Roasted Vegetable Soup with Parmesan Cheese 140

Yellow Lentil Dip with Olives and Red Peppers 141

Chia Cacao Pudding 142

Ricotta à la Méditerranée 143

Baked Mixed Fruit with Cinnamon 144

Mango Lime Mousse 145

Mixed Dried Fruit with Parmesan Cheese

Gluten-Free Vegetarian	Prep time: 5 minutes Serves: 1

Who doesn't like to snack on cheese or fruit? This recipe brings these two favorites together for a delectable flavor combination. And dried fruit is still as nutritious as fresh! Even though the water has been removed, it still contains all of the nutrients, fiber, and antioxidants of the fresh variety. Just be sure to choose dried fruits that have no added sugars on the ingredients list.

2 dried figs, sliced

2 dried apricots, sliced

2 prunes, sliced

1 ounce chunk Parmesan cheese, sliced

1. In a bowl, mix all the ingredients well.

2. Store leftovers in a sealed container in the refrigerator for up to 4 days.

> **Swap and substitute:** Even though this recipe calls for two of each type of fruit, if you want to use exclusively one fruit in the same quantities, that will also work. However, don't swap the cheese—Parmesan has less fat and fewer calories than most other cheeses.

Per serving: Calories: 215; Fat: 7.5g; Carbohydrates: 28g; Fiber: 3.5g; Sugar: 19g; Protein: 11g; Sodium: 393mg

Mini Parfait

Gluten-Free Vegetarian	**Prep time:** 5 minutes **Serves:** 1

This is the perfect 3 or 4 p.m. pick-me-up snack, because it contains healthy carbohydrates for energy to get you through the afternoon and protein to keep you satiated until dinner. When it comes to weight loss, an afternoon snack can save you from overeating at dinner. Choose whatever berries you like best for this recipe.

½ cup plain 2% Greek yogurt

¾ cup frozen berries, thawed (or fresh)

1 teaspoon honey

1 tablespoon chopped walnuts

1. Spoon the yogurt into a small glass container.

2. Layer the berries on top of the yogurt, drizzle with honey, and top with the walnuts before enjoying.

Make it easy: You can make a few of these ahead of time, store them in sealed 8-ounce containers in the refrigerator for up to 4 days, and eat them throughout the week.

Per serving: Calories: 204; Fat: 8g; Carbohydrates: 24g; Fiber: 3.5g; Sugar: 18g; Protein: 14g; Sodium: 42mg

Applesauce with Seeds

Dairy-Free Gluten-Free Vegan	**Prep time:** 5 minutes **Serves:** 1

This light, yet fulfilling snack provides good fats, fiber, and protein from the seeds. Chia seeds and flaxseed in particular contain plant-based omega-3s, which are great anti-inflammatory fats. The smooth texture of the applesauce contrasts nicely with the crunch of the seeds.

½ cup unsweetened
   applesauce

1 teaspoon chia seeds

1 teaspoon sesame seeds

1 teaspoon flaxseed

1 teaspoon raw
   pumpkin seeds

1. In a small bowl, sprinkle the seeds on top of the applesauce. Mix well if desired.

2. Store leftovers in a sealed container in the refrigerator for up to 4 days.

Swap or substitute: Don't have all of the seeds listed on hand? You can stick with just 1 or 2 types of seeds in the same quantities.

Per serving: Calories: 123; Fat: 5.5g; Carbohydrates: 17g; Fiber: 4g; Sugar: 11g; Protein: 3g; Sodium: 10mg

Hard-Boiled Egg and Apple Slices

Dairy-Free Gluten-Free Vegetarian	**Prep time:** 5 minutes **Cook time:** 10 minutes **Serves:** 1

There are many different ways to hard-boil an egg. This recipe details how I've been making mine for years. This portable snack is the perfect combo of complex carbs, fat, and protein that you can make ahead of time and have on hand all week.

2 large eggs

1 medium apple, sliced

1. In a small pot, place the eggs in a single layer and cover them with cold water. Bring the water to a boil.

2. Start a timer for 7 minutes, then remove the pot from the heat. Drain the eggs and place them immediately in a bowl of ice water. Peel once cooled.

3. Enjoy immediately, or place the apple slices and eggs in a zip-top bag or sealable container.

> **Store it:** If storing them or taking them to go, you can squeeze some lemon juice on the apple to prevent it from browning. Hard-boiled eggs will hold in a sealed container in the refrigerator for up to 3 days.

Per serving: **Calories: 238**; Fat: 10g; Carbohydrates: 26g; Fiber: 4.5g; Sugar: 19g; Protein: 13g; Sodium: 144mg

Mason Jar Roasted Vegetable Soup with Parmesan Cheese

Gluten-Free	Prep time: 5 minutes / Cook time: 90 seconds / Serves: 1

On colder afternoons, I like something savory and comforting. When I recommend this to clients as a snack, they report that they love it. There's nothing like this delicious soup in a Mason jar with a little cheese on top. This recipe is a great way to use up leftover roasted veggies.

1½ cups Roasted Vegetables (page 154)

1 cup low-sodium chicken or vegetable broth

1 tablespoon shredded Parmesan cheese

1. In a blender, combine the roasted vegetables and broth and blend well.

2. Pour into a jar and sprinkle cheese on top. Heat in the microwave for 90 seconds and enjoy, or cover and refrigerate for later.

Make it easy: Prepare several servings in advance for the week and store in sealed containers in the refrigerator for up to 4 days for a warming grab-and-go snack.

Per serving: Calories: 115; Fat: 4g; Carbohydrates: 14g; Fiber: 4.5g; Sugar: 5g; Protein: 7g; Sodium: 788mg

Yellow Lentil Dip with Olives and Red Peppers

Dairy-Free Gluten-Free Vegan	Prep time: 5 minutes Serves: 1

If you like hummus, you will love this yellow lentil dip, especially dressed up with olives and red peppers. The dip has the same mouthfeel that hits the spot without all the calories, making it another great savory snack to enjoy between meals. Rice crackers are a nice low-cal vessel for the dip and are readily available in grocery stores.

¼ cup Yellow Lentil Dip (page 157)

4 kalamata olives, chopped

2 tablespoons diced red bell peppers

5 rice crackers

1. In a small bowl, sprinkle the lentil dip with the olives and red peppers.

2. Enjoy with rice crackers.

3. Store leftovers in a sealed container in the refrigerator for up to 4 days.

Swap or substitute: If gluten isn't an issue, you can replace the rice crackers with low-fat whole-grain crackers. You can also use this as a dip for any of your favorite crunchy vegetables, such as celery, cauliflower, or cherry tomatoes.

Per serving: Calories: 257; Fat: 11g; Carbohydrates: 32g; Fiber: 4g; Sugar: 2g; Protein: 9g; Sodium: 676mg

Chia Cacao Pudding

Gluten-Free Vegetarian	Prep time: 10 minutes, plus 6 hours to set Serves: 2

Listen up, chocolate lovers: This pudding will not only satisfy your sweet tooth, but it'll also reward you with the antioxidants from the cacao. As a bonus, the chia seeds expand when in liquids, making you feel fuller.

1 cup 1% milk

3 tablespoons chia seeds

1 tablespoon
   cacao powder

½ teaspoon stevia

1. In a jar or small to-go container, mix all the ingredients until well combined.

2. Refrigerate for at least 6 hours up to overnight to thicken before enjoying.

Store it: Store leftovers in sealed individual containers in the refrigerator for up to 3 days.

Per serving: **Calories: 144**; Fat: 6.5g; Carbohydrates: 14g; Fiber: 5.5g; Sugar: 6g; Protein: 7g; Sodium: 56mg

Ricotta à la Méditerranée

Gluten-Free **Vegetarian**	**Prep time:** 5 minutes **Serves:** 1

This quick dessert will send your taste buds straight to the Mediterranean. Ricotta cheese is overlooked in low-calorie eating, but it's really great for desserts. Here we'll use part-skim cheese, which is lower in fat and calories.

½ cup part-skim
  ricotta cheese

1 teaspoon
  chopped walnuts

1 dried fig, sliced

1 teaspoon honey

Ground cinnamon

1. In a small bowl, layer the walnuts and fig slices on top of the ricotta.

2. Drizzle with honey and sprinkle with cinnamon before enjoying.

3. Store leftovers in a sealed container in the refrigerator for up to 3 days.

> **Swap or substitute:** You can use 2% milkfat cottage cheese instead in the same quantity.

Per serving: Calories: 229; Fat: 11g; Carbohydrates: 18g; Fiber: 1g; Sugar: 10g; Protein: 15g; Sodium: 124mg

Baked Mixed Fruit with Cinnamon

Dairy-Free Gluten-Free Vegan	**Prep time:** 15 minutes **Cook time:** 35 minutes **Serves:** 12

This dessert eats just like a pie without the crust. The combination of sour and sweet fruit with a touch of sea salt to enhance the flavor will have your family singing your praises after supper. It's low in calories as well as delicious, making it a winning dessert.

Nonstick cooking spray

1 pound apple wedges

8 ounces
   pineapple wedges

8 ounces mango strips

8 ounces peach wedges

6 ounces (about 2)
   Sungold kiwi wedges

⅛ teaspoon sea
   salt, divided

2 tablespoons
   brown sugar

2 teaspoons ground
   cinnamon

1. Preheat the oven to 400°F. Spray an 11-by-8-inch baking dish with nonstick spray.

2. In a bowl, mix together the apples, pineapple, mangos, peaches, and kiwi. In the bottom of the prepared baking dish, arrange the first layer of the fruit. Sprinkle a layer of sea salt over the first layer of fruit, then repeat two more times so you have three layers of fruit.

3. Sprinkle the brown sugar evenly on the top layer. Bake uncovered for 35 minutes. Sprinkle with cinnamon before serving. Store leftovers in a sealed container in the refrigerator for up to 4 days.

Swap or substitute: You can also use canned peaches or pineapple. Just make sure they are in their own juices, not syrup.

Per serving (1 cup): Calories: 75; Fat: 1.5g; Carbohydrates: 17g; Fiber: 2g; Sugar: 14g; Protein: 1g; Sodium: 26mg

Mango Lime Mousse

Gluten-Free Vegetarian	**Prep time:** 10 minutes, plus 4 hours to chill **Serves:** 4

This recipe started as an idea for a key lime pie and ended up as a mousse—it's just as sweetly satisfying. This recipe uses monk fruit, a natural sugar alcohol that's made from fruit and contains no calories.

1 mango, peeled and cut into chunks

8 ounces ⅓-less-fat cream cheese (Neufchâtel)

¼ cup lime juice

2 tablespoons monk fruit sweetener

1. In a food processor or small blender, blend the mango until smooth.

2. In a bowl, combine the mango purée, cream cheese, lime juice, and sweetener. Using a hand mixer, blend until combined.

3. Cover and chill in the refrigerator for 4 hours before enjoying. Store leftovers in a sealed container in the refrigerator for up to 3 days.

Per serving (½ cup): Calories: 197; Fat: 12g; Carbohydrates: 17g; Fiber: 1.5g; Sugar: 14g; Protein: 5g; Sodium: 241mg

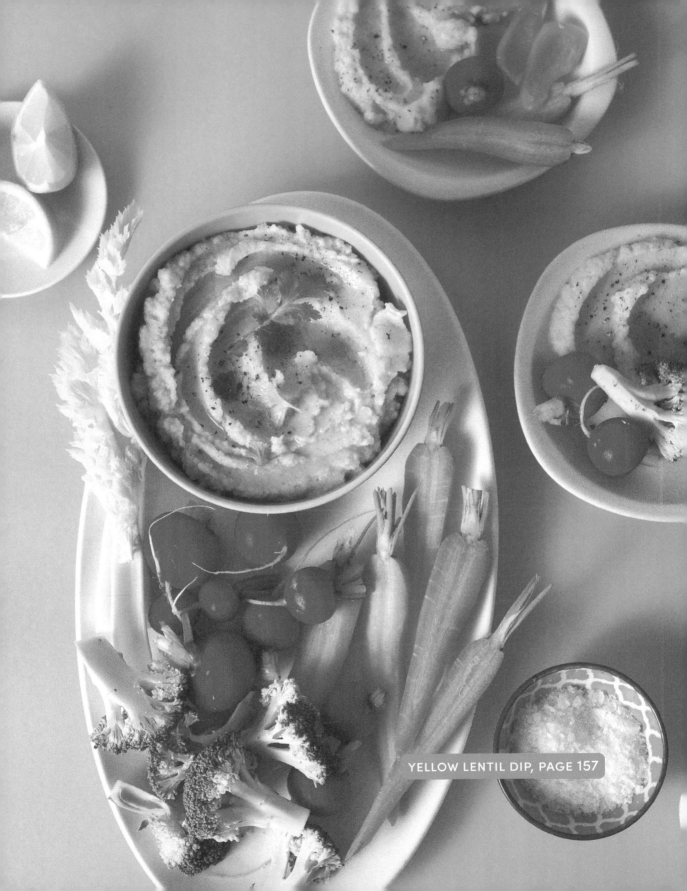

YELLOW LENTIL DIP, PAGE 157

CHAPTER EIGHT

KITCHEN STAPLES, DRESSINGS, AND SAUCES

Roasted Chicken 148

Basic Farro 149

Basic Brown Rice 150

Basic Flavorful Quinoa 151

Steamed Broccoli and Cauliflower with Lemon Juice 152

Roasted Vegetables 154

Lemon-Mustard Vinaigrette 155

Cilantro-Infused Yogurt Dressing 156

Yellow Lentil Dip 157

Mixed Berries Sweet Sauce 158

Roasted Chicken

Dairy-Free **Gluten-Free**	**Prep time:** 10 minutes / **Cook time:** 10 minutes / **Serves:** 4

This cooked chicken recipe can be used in many other recipes in this book and for grain bowls and salads. Roasting is a fast cooking method that can help keep chicken breasts juicy and healthy with little added oil. You want to make sure the poultry doesn't overcook—a timer will help you come out with perfectly cooked chicken for the week.

Nonstick cooking spray

1 pound boneless, skinless
  chicken breasts

1 teaspoon sea salt

½ teaspoon freshly
  ground black pepper

1. Preheat the oven to 500°F. Spray a 9-by-13-inch baking dish or a large roasting pan with cooking spray and set aside.

2. On a cutting board, butterfly the chicken. Do this by placing your hand on top of the breast and using a chef's knife to slice into one side of the breast lengthwise, starting at the thicker end and ending at the thin point. Be careful not to cut all the way through to the other side.

3. In the baking dish, place the chicken breasts in a single layer with the sides folded out like a butterfly. Spray more oil on top of the breasts and season them with salt and pepper.

4. Bake the chicken for 12 minutes. Remove from the oven and let sit for 5 minutes.

Store it: Cooled roasted chicken can be stored in an airtight container in the refrigerator for up to 4 days.

Per serving (3 ounces cooked): Calories: 133; Fat: 3.5g; Carbohydrates: 0g; Fiber: 0g; Sugar: 0g; Protein: 23g; Sodium: 637mg

Basic Farro

Dairy-Free	Prep time: 5 minutes / Cook time: 40 minutes / Serves: 6

Farro is the wheat of Italy, so it's only appropriate that it cooks like pasta in a sense rather than rice. This ancient grain offers lots of antioxidants and plenty of fiber to keep your heart healthy and your belly full. Pair this grain with anything you'd serve with rice.

1 cup dry farro

1 teaspoon canola oil

¼ cup diced yellow onion

¼ teaspoon chopped garlic

3 cups water or vegetable or chicken broth

½ teaspoon sea salt

1. In a sieve, rinse the farro under cold water until the water runs clear. Set aside.

2. In a small pot over medium heat, heat the oil and sauté the onion for 3 minutes or until translucent. Add the garlic and sauté for another minute.

3. Add the water, farro, and salt to the pot and bring to a boil. Cover and reduce heat to low. Simmer until the farro is soft, 35 to 40 minutes.

4. Using the sieve, drain the extra water. With a fork, fluff the farro before serving.

Store it: Store leftover farro in a sealed container in the refrigerator for up to 4 days.

Per serving (½ cup): Calories: 116; Fat: 0.5g; Carbohydrates: 23g; Fiber: 2g; Sugar: 0g; Protein: 5g; Sodium: 117mg

Basic Brown Rice

Dairy-Free Gluten-Free	Prep time: 5 minutes Cook time: 45 minutes Serves: 6

Brown rice is a wonderful whole grain that makes a versatile side or base and keeps you full for hours. You can always just steam or boil brown rice, but I wanted to make it more fun and flavorful without adding additional calories by including onion and garlic in this classic staple.

1 cup dry brown rice

1 teaspoon canola oil

¼ cup diced yellow onion

¼ teaspoon
  chopped garlic

1 medium red bell pepper

2½ cups water or chicken
  or vegetable broth

½ teaspoon sea salt

1. In a sieve, rinse the brown rice under cold water until the water runs clear. Set aside.

2. In a small pot over medium heat, heat the oil and sauté the onion for 3 minutes. Add the garlic and bell pepper and sauté for another minute, or until fragrant.

3. Add the water, rice, and salt to the pot and bring to a boil. Cover and reduce heat to low. Simmer until all the water is absorbed, about 40 minutes. Fluff the brown rice with a fork.

> **Store it:** Store leftovers in a sealed container in the refrigerator for up to 4 days.

Per serving (½ cup): **Calories:** 129; **Fat:** 2g; **Carbohydrates:** 25g; **Fiber:** 1.5g; **Sugar:** 1.5g; **Protein:** 3g; **Sodium:** 196mg

Basic Flavorful Quinoa

Dairy-Free Gluten-Free	Prep time: 5 minutes Cook time: 15 minutes Serves: 6

Quinoa has gained some traction in the health world as of late, but many people ask how they can make it tastier. There are lots of flavorful quinoa dishes, but even with this recipe, you can elevate your quinoa and add it to your proteins and veggies for a complete meal.

1 teaspoon extra-virgin olive oil

¼ cup chopped yellow onion

1 cup white quinoa

1¾ cups water or chicken or vegetable broth

½ teaspoon sea salt

1 teaspoon tomato paste

1. In a 4-quart pot over medium heat, heat the oil for about 1 minute. Add the onion and sauté for about 2 minutes, or until soft.

2. Meanwhile, in a sieve, rinse the quinoa under cold water until the water runs clear. Transfer it to the pot. Stir in the water, salt, and tomato paste.

3. Bring to a boil, cover, and reduce heat to low. Simmer until all the water is absorbed, 15 to 20 minutes. With a fork, fluff the quinoa.

Store it: Store leftovers in a sealed container in the refrigerator for up to 3 days.

Per serving (½ cup): **Calories:** 123; **Fat:** 1.5g; **Carbohydrates:** 23g; **Fiber:** 2g; **Sugar:** 2.5g; **Protein:** 4g; **Sodium:** 200mg

Steamed Broccoli and Cauliflower with Lemon Juice

Gluten-Free **Dairy-Free** **Vegan**	**Prep time:** 10 minutes **Cook time:** 5 minutes **Serves:** 4

The perfect seasoning for steamed broccoli and cauliflower is, quite simply, sea salt and lemon juice. They are common and inexpensive, yet they bring out the flavor in your vegetables with gusto—and none of the added calories.

½ head (3½ cups) broccoli florets

½ head (3½ cups) cauliflower florets

2 tablespoons lemon juice

1 tablespoon extra-virgin olive oil

½ teaspoon sea salt

STOVETOP

1. In a 4-quart pot, bring 1 to 2 inches of water to a boil. Add the broccoli and cauliflower to the pot and cover.

2. Cook for 3 to 4 minutes, or until semisoft. Place the vegetables in a colander and rinse with cold water.

3. Season with the lemon juice, oil, and salt. Store leftovers in a sealed container in the refrigerator for up to 2 days.

MICROWAVE

1. Wash the broccoli and cauliflower and leave them wet. In a large bowl, loosely cover the broccoli and cauliflower with a lid or a microwave cover.

2. Microwave on high for 3 to 4 minutes, or until tender. Place the vegetables in a colander and rinse with cold water.

3. Season with the lemon juice, oil, and salt. Store leftovers in a sealed container in the refrigerator for up to 2 days.

Bulk it up: I love having steamed vegetables on hand—you can snack on them to shoo away that pre-meal hunger while you cook, rather than reaching for chips or cookies.

Per serving (1½ cups): Calories: 72; Fat: 4g; Carbohydrates: 8g; Fiber: 3.5g; Sugar: 3g; Protein: 4g, Sodium: 336mg

Roasted Vegetables

Gluten-Free Dairy-Free Vegan	**Prep time:** 10 minutes **Cook time:** 20 minutes **Serves:** 6

If there's one way I have convinced my clients to eat more vegetables, it's by encouraging them to roast them. Roasting veggies brings out their natural sugars and flavors, giving them a different and very enjoyable flavor profile. You'll only want to eat vegetables this way for the rest of your life.

2 cups Brussels sprouts

1 head cauliflower, chopped into florets

1 medium red onion

1 medium bell pepper

1 (8-inch) zucchini

1 (6-inch) carrot

1 tablespoon extra-virgin olive oil

1½ teaspoons sea salt

½ teaspoon freshly ground black pepper

½ teaspoon garlic powder

1. Preheat the oven to 450°F.

2. Chop all the vegetables into pieces of equivalent size, 1 to 2 inches.

3. In a roasting pan, place the vegetables, add the oil, and season with the salt, pepper, and garlic powder. Toss to fully coat the vegetables.

4. Cook for 20 minutes or until tender and the edges are browned. Store leftovers in a sealed container in the refrigerator for up to 4 days.

Make it easy: After 3 days, roasted vegetables begin to wilt and gradually lose the crisp, flavorful appeal on their own. Luckily, this is the best time to use them in your Mason Jar Roasted Vegetable Soup with Parmesan Cheese (page 140). That way, you don't have to waste any food and can get a killer snack out of the leftovers.

Per serving (1½ cups): **Calories:** 79; **Fat:** 3g; **Carbohydrates:** 12g; **Fiber:** 4.5g; **Sugar:** 5g; **Protein:** 4g; **Sodium:** 628mg

Lemon-Mustard Vinaigrette

Gluten-Free Dairy-Free Vegan	**Prep time:** 5 minutes, plus 10 minutes to sit **Makes:** ¾ cup

This is a deliciously light salad dressing that's easy to make with ingredients you're likely to have on hand, so if you need to throw together a dressing in a pinch, this is the recipe for you.

½ cup lemon juice

2 teaspoons
   yellow mustard

¼ teaspoon freshly
   ground black pepper

½ teaspoon dried basil

½ teaspoon sea salt

2 tablespoons extra-virgin
   olive oil

1. In a small bowl, whisk together all the ingredients until well blended.

2. Let sit for 10 minutes. Enjoy right away or refrigerate for later, making sure to stir well before each use.

Store it: Store dressing in a sealed container in the refrigerator for up to 4 days.

Per serving (2 tablespoons): **Calories: 45**; Fat: 4.5g; Carbohydrates: 1g; Fiber: 0g; Sugar: 0.5g; Protein: 0g; Sodium: 212mg

Cilantro-Infused Yogurt Dressing

Gluten-Free **Vegetarian**	**Prep time:** 10 minutes, plus 10 minutes to sit **Makes:** 1½ cups

Ranch dressing, move aside! This recipe is going to replace your creamy dressings as your favorite salad topping, as it delivers all the creaminess you crave without all the saturated fat and extra calories.

1 cup plain
  2% Greek yogurt

⅓ cup avocado oil
  mayonnaise

2 tablespoons lemon juice

½ cup finely chopped
  cilantro leaves

½ teaspoon minced garlic

½ teaspoon sea salt

¼ teaspoon freshly
  ground black pepper

1. In a small bowl, whisk together all the ingredients until well blended.

2. Let sit for 10 minutes. Enjoy right away or refrigerate for later, making sure to stir well before each use.

Store it: Store dressing in a sealed container in the refrigerator for up to 4 days.

Per serving (3 tablespoons): Calories: 90; Fat: 8.5g; Carbohydrates: 2g; Fiber: 0g; Sugar: 1g; Protein: 3g; Sodium: 240mg

Yellow Lentil Dip

Dairy-Free Gluten-Free Vegan	**Prep time:** 10 minutes **Cook time:** 15 minutes **Makes:** 1 cup

Traditional hummus uses chickpeas, but this recipe calls for lentils instead. It's still creamy without all the calories, and makes a perfect dip for veggies, or a spread for wraps and sandwiches. Garnish with fresh cilantro, if desired.

½ cup dry yellow lentils

1½ cups water

2 tablespoons lemon juice

1½ tablespoons
  extra-virgin olive oil

½ teaspoon sea salt

¼ teaspoon freshly
  ground black pepper

⅛ teaspoon garlic powder

1. Bring a small saucepan of water to a boil. Add the lentils and cook for 5 to 10 minutes, until tender.

2. Drain the lentils and transfer to a blender. Add the 1½ cups water, lemon juice, olive oil, salt, pepper, and garlic powder and blend until you reach a smooth consistency.

Store it: Store in a sealed container in the refrigerator for up to 3 days.

Per serving (¼ cup): **Calories:** 136; Fat: 5.5g; Carbohydrates: 16g; Fiber: 2.5g; Sugar: 1g; Protein: 7g; Sodium: 292mg

Mixed Berries Sweet Sauce

Dairy-Free Gluten-Free Vegan	Prep time: 10 minutes Cook time: 35 minutes Makes: 2 cups

You'll forget that maple syrup in your pantry after you try this sauce on your pancakes or waffles. This delicious sauce uses frozen fruit (mixed berries of your choice), so you can get your fruit servings in while enjoying a treat. It's a win-win!

4 cups frozen mixed
   berries, thawed

1 cup water

3 cloves

2 cinnamon sticks

Peel of one
   orange, washed

¾ cup monk fruit
   sweetener

1. In a sieve, run warm water over the frozen berries for about 1 minute or until defrosted.

2. Add the fruit to a blender with the water and blend until you reach a smooth consistency.

3. In a small saucepan, combine the berry blend with the rest of the ingredients and bring to a boil, stirring occasionally.

4. Simmer the sauce until it is thick and has reduced by half.

5. Let it cool. Press the sauce through a sieve so only the juice remains, and store in a jar with a tight seal.

Store it: Store in a sealed container in the refrigerator for up to 5 days.

Per serving (2 tablespoons): Calories: 19; Fat: 0g; Carbohydrates: 5g; Fiber: 1g; Sugar: 3.5g; Protein: 0g; Sodium: 0mg

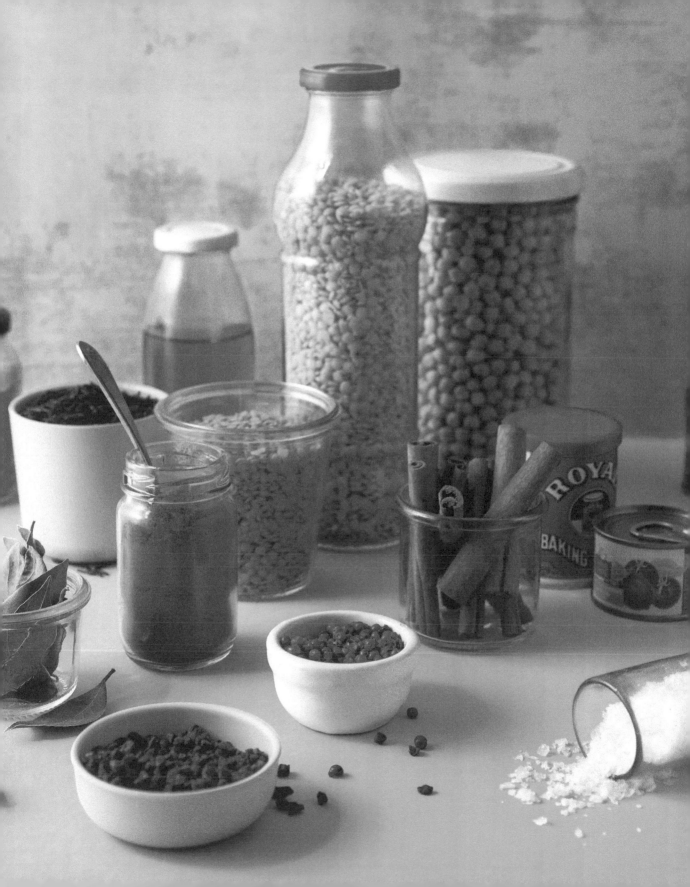

Measurement Conversions

VOLUME EQUIVALENTS	U.S. STANDARD	U.S. STANDARD (OUNCES)	METRIC (APPROXIMATE)
LIQUID	2 tablespoons	1 fl. oz.	30 mL
	¼ cup	2 fl. oz.	60 mL
	½ cup	4 fl. oz.	120 mL
	1 cup	8 fl. oz.	240 mL
	1½ cups	12 fl. oz.	355 mL
	2 cups or 1 pint	16 fl. oz.	475 mL
	4 cups or 1 quart	32 fl. oz.	1 L
	1 gallon	128 fl. oz.	4 L
DRY	⅛ teaspoon	—	0.5 mL
	¼ teaspoon	—	1 mL
	½ teaspoon	—	2 mL
	¾ teaspoon	—	4 mL
	1 teaspoon	—	5 mL
	1 tablespoon	—	15 mL
	¼ cup	—	59 mL
	⅓ cup	—	79 mL
	½ cup	—	118 mL
	⅔ cup	—	156 mL
	¾ cup	—	177 mL
	1 cup	—	235 mL
	2 cups or 1 pint	—	475 mL
	3 cups	—	700 mL
	4 cups or 1 quart	—	1 L
	½ gallon	—	2 L
	1 gallon	—	4 L

OVEN TEMPERATURES

FAHRENHEIT	CELSIUS (APPROXIMATE)
250°F	120°C
300°F	150°C
325°F	165°C
350°F	180°C
375°F	190°C
400°F	200°C
425°F	220°C
450°F	230°C

WEIGHT EQUIVALENTS

U.S. STANDARD	METRIC (APPROXIMATE)
½ ounce	15 g
1 ounce	30 g
2 ounces	60 g
4 ounces	115 g
8 ounces	225 g
12 ounces	340 g
16 ounces or 1 pound	455 g

Resources

AUTHOR WEBSITE

Visit ManuelVillacorta.com for articles, recipes, other published work, and more.

CALORIE COUNTERS

There are many free online calorie counters, including one at a website Manuel founded, Whole Body Reboot. With a free seven-day trial, you can use this calculator, which not only gives you your energy expenditure for the day but also how much you should be eating based on your body statistics. You can find this calculator at WholeBodyReboot.com.

FURTHER READING ON MSG

ManuelVillacorta.com/2020/03/30/the-culinary-benefits-of-msg-with-health-and-flavor

ManuelVillacorta.com/2018/10/09/what-you-need-to-know-about-msg-a-series

DESTINI MOODY

Moody, a certified personal trainer and board-certified sports dietitian, provided the exercise recommendations and content in chapter 2 of this book. You can find her on social media—on Twitter (@TheAthletesRD) and Instagram (@TheAthletesDietitian)—or at her website, TheAthletesDietitian.com.

References

Macpherson, R. E., T. J. Hazell, T. D. Olver, D. H. Paterson, and P. W. Lemon. "Run Sprint Interval Training Improves Aerobic Performance but Not Maximal Cardiac Output." *Medicine and Science in Sports and Exercise* 43, no. 1 (2011): 115–122. doi.org/10.1249/MSS.0b013e3181e5eacd.

Mattes, Richard D. "Hunger and Thirst: Issues in Measurement and Prediction of Eating and Drinking." *Science Direct.* January 11, 2010. doi.org/10.1016/j.physbeh.2009.12.026.

Moody, Destini. "Often Feeling Hungry? You May Just Be Thirsty." *Manuel Villacorta.* July 24, 2017. ManuelVillacorta.com/2017/07/24/often-feeling-hungry-you-may-just-be-thirsty.

Trapp, E. G., D. J. Chisholm, J. Freund, and S. H. Boutcher. "The Effects of High-Intensity Intermittent Exercise Training on Fat Loss and Fasting Insulin Levels of Young Women." *International Journal of Obesity* 32, no. 4 (2008): 684–691. doi.org/10.1038/sj.ijo.0803781.

Tremblay, A., J. A. Simoneau, and C. Bouchard. "Impact of Exercise Intensity on Body Fatness and Skeletal Muscle Metabolism." *Metabolism: Clinical and Experimental* 43, no. 7 (1994): 814–818. doi.org/10.1016/0026-0495(94)90259-3.

Treuth, M. S., G. R. Hunter, and M. Williams. "Effects of Exercise Intensity on 24-h Energy Expenditure and Substrate Oxidation." *Medicine and Science in Sports and Exercise* 28, no. 9 (1996): 1138–1143. doi.org/10.1097/00005768-199609000-00009.

Index

A

Accountability, 8
Apples
  Baked Mixed Fruit with Cinnamon, 144
  Chicken Apple Salad, 82
  Hard-Boiled Egg and Apple Slices, 139
Applesauce
  Applesauce with Seeds, 138
  Warm Apple-Spiced Smoothie, 54
Asparagus, Sheet Pan Glazed Balsamic
    Salmon with Asparagus, 105
Avocados
  Avocado, Tomato, and Poached
    Egg Toast, 78
  Citrus Quinoa Avocado Salad
    with Roasted Chicken, 83
  Creamy Green Smoothie, 57
  Egg and Avocado Burritos, 70–71

B

Baked Mixed Fruit with Cinnamon, 144
Banana Cacao Oat Pancakes, 67
Basal metabolic rate (BMR), 10
Basic Brown Rice, 150
Basic Farro, 149
Basic Flavorful Quinoa, 151
Beans
  Black Bean, Corn, and Chicken
    Sausage Bowl, 98
  Blackened Fish with Bean Salad, 104
  Electric Pressure Cooker Chicken,
    White Beans, Spinach, and
    Mushrooms in White Wine, 122–123
Beef
  Beef and Vegetable Stir-Fry, 121
  Electric Pressure Cooker Low-Cal
    Beef Bourguignon, 124–125
  Lean Beef Meatballs in Tomato
    Sauce with Polenta, 128–129
  Roast Beef and Cheese Panini, 79

Bell peppers
  Glazed Pork Tenderloin and
    Bell Peppers, 130–131
  Ground Turkey and Vegetable
    Stuffed Bell Peppers, 118–119
  Yellow Lentil Dip with Olives
    and Red Peppers, 141
Berries
  Berry Mango Bliss Smoothie, 56
  Cacao Coconut Cranberry Quinoa
    Breakfast Bowl, 61
  High-Protein Overnight Oats, 60
  Mini Parfait, 137
  Mixed Berries Sweet Sauce, 158
  Superfood Parfait, 58
Black Bean, Corn, and Chicken
    Sausage Bowl, 98
Blackened Fish with Bean Salad, 104
Bowls
  Black Bean, Corn, and Chicken
    Sausage Bowl, 98
  Cacao Coconut Cranberry Quinoa
    Breakfast Bowl, 61
  Chicken Pomodoro Farro Bowl, 99
Bread, Butternut Squash Walnut, 74–75
Broccoli and Cauliflower, Steamed,
    with Lemon Juice, 152–153
Burritos, Egg and Avocado, 70–71
Butternut squash
  Butternut Squash Walnut Bread, 74–75
  Sheet Pan Mediterranean Chicken
    with Butternut Squash, 109

C

Cacao nibs
  Banana Cacao Oat Pancakes, 67
  Cacao Coconut Cranberry Quinoa
    Breakfast Bowl, 61
  Chia Cacao Pudding, 142
  Superfood Parfait, 58

California-Style Scrambled Eggs, 63
Calorie calculators, 10
Calorie needs, 9–10
Calories, 3–5, 6, 20
Caramelized Onions and Spinach with
    Glazed Balsamic Salmon, 87–88
Cardio exercise, 18
Cauliflower
  Light Farfalle and Cheese with
      Cauliflower, 96–97
  Sheet Pan Roasted Tofu and
      Cauliflower, 106–107
  Steamed Broccoli and Cauliflower
      with Lemon Juice, 152–153
Cheese
  Egg, Cheese, and Ham English
      Muffins, 68–69
  Light Farfalle and Cheese with
      Cauliflower, 96–97
  Mason Jar Roasted Vegetable Soup
      with Parmesan Cheese, 140
  Mixed Dried Fruit with
      Parmesan Cheese, 136
  Ricotta à la Méditerranée, 143
  Roast Beef and Cheese Panini, 79
  Vegetable-Layered Cheese Lasagna, 127
Chia seeds
  Applesauce with Seeds, 138
  Chia Cacao Pudding, 142
  Dried Fruit and Chia High-
      Protein Muffins, 72–73
Chicken
  Black Bean, Corn, and Chicken
      Sausage Bowl, 98
  Chicken and Potato Salad with
      Yogurt Dressing, 92
  Chicken Apple Salad, 82
  Chicken Cilantro Patties, 89
  Chicken Pomodoro Farro Bowl, 99
  Citrus Quinoa Avocado Salad
      with Roasted Chicken, 83
  Curried Chicken Pita Wraps, 81
  Electric Pressure Cooker Chicken,
      White Beans, Spinach, and
      Mushrooms in White Wine, 122–123

  Mayo-Yogurt Baked Chicken with
      Mini Potatoes, 116–117
  Peruvian-Style Arroz con Pollo, 113–114
  Roasted Chicken, 148
  Sheet Pan Mediterranean Chicken
      with Butternut Squash, 109
  Wild Fiesta Rice with Roasted Chicken, 115
Chickpeas
  Chickpea Stir-Fry, 120
  Tomato Chickpea Soup, 93
Cilantro
  Chicken Cilantro Patties, 89
  Cilantro-Infused Yogurt Dressing, 156
Citrus Quinoa Avocado Salad with
    Roasted Chicken, 83
Coconut Cacao Cranberry Quinoa
    Breakfast Bowl, 61
Core exercises
  flutter kicks, 29
  high plank, 28
  mountain climbers, 30
Corn, Black Bean, and Chicken
    Sausage Bowl, 98
Creamy Green Smoothie, 57
Crustless Egg and Spinach Quiches, 66
Curried Chicken Pita Wraps, 81

D

Dairy-free
  Applesauce with Seeds, 138
  Avocado, Tomato, and Poached
      Egg Toast, 78
  Baked Mixed Fruit with Cinnamon, 144
  Basic Brown Rice, 150
  Basic Farro, 149
  Basic Flavorful Quinoa, 151
  Beef and Vegetable Stir-Fry, 121
  Black Bean, Corn, and Chicken
      Sausage Bowl, 98
  Blackened Fish with Bean Salad, 104
  California-Style Scrambled Eggs, 63
  Caramelized Onions and Spinach with
      Glazed Balsamic Salmon, 87–88
  Chicken Cilantro Patties, 89
  Chicken Pomodoro Farro Bowl, 99

Chickpea Stir-Fry, 120
Electric Pressure Cooker Chicken,
    White Beans, Spinach, and
    Mushrooms in White Wine, 122–123
Electric Pressure Cooker Low-Cal
    Beef Bourguignon, 124–125
Electric Pressure Cooker Red
    Lentil Soup, 126
Fish Tacos with Mango and Kiwi Salsa, 84
Fried Shrimp Brown Rice, 110
Glazed Pork Tenderloin and
    Bell Peppers, 130–131
Ground Pork Endive Cups, 85
Ground Turkey and Vegetable
    Stuffed Bell Peppers, 118–119
Hard-Boiled Egg and Apple Slices, 139
Lemon-Mustard Vinaigrette, 155
Mixed Berries Sweet Sauce, 158
Peruvian-Style Arroz con Pollo, 113–114
Roasted Chicken, 148
Roasted Vegetables, 154
Seafood à la Paella with Farro, 111
Sheet Pan Glazed Balsamic Salmon
    with Asparagus, 105
Sheet Pan Mediterranean Chicken
    with Butternut Squash, 109
Sheet Pan Roasted Tofu and
    Cauliflower, 106–107
Shrimp and Vegetable Wild
    Rice Bowl, 100–101
Steamed Broccoli and Cauliflower
    with Lemon Juice, 152–153
Sun-Dried Tomato and Vegetable
    Frittata, 64–65
Tomato Chickpea Soup, 93
Turkey Meatball Quinoa Soup, 94–95
Wild Fiesta Rice with Roasted Chicken, 115
Yellow Lentil Dip, 157
Yellow Lentil Dip with Olives
    and Red Peppers, 141
Dairy products. *See also specific*
Desserts
Baked Mixed Fruit with Cinnamon, 144
Chia Cacao Pudding, 142
Mango Lime Mousse, 145
Ricotta à la Méditerranée, 143

Dips
Yellow Lentil Dip, 157
Yellow Lentil Dip with Olives
    and Red Peppers, 141
Dressings
Cilantro-Infused Yogurt Dressing, 156
Lemon-Mustard Vinaigrette, 155
Dried Fruit and Chia High-
    Protein Muffins, 72–73

E

Eggs
Avocado, Tomato, and Poached
    Egg Toast, 78
California-Style Scrambled Eggs, 63
Crustless Egg and Spinach
    Quiches, 66
Egg and Avocado Burritos, 70–71
Egg, Cheese, and Ham English
    Muffins, 68–69
Hard-Boiled Egg and Apple
    Slices, 139
Sheet Pan Cracked-Egg Pizza, 108
Sun-Dried Tomato and Vegetable
    Frittata, 64–65
Umami Scrambled Eggs, 62
Electric Pressure Cooker Chicken, White
    Beans, Spinach, and Mushrooms
    in White Wine, 122–123
Electric Pressure Cooker Low-Cal
    Beef Bourguignon, 124–125
Electric Pressure Cooker Red
    Lentil Soup, 126
Empty calories, 4, 9
Endive Cups, Ground Pork, 85
English Muffins, Egg, Cheese,
    and Ham, 68–69
Exercise
benefits of, 16
cardio, 18
core, 28–30
dangers of overexercising, 17
importance of, 8
lower body, 21–23
myths, 19
recovery days, 19–20

Exercise (*continued*)
  routine-setting, 17–18
  strength/resistance training, 18
  upper body, 24–27
  workout plan, 31

F

Farro
  Basic Farro, 149
  Chicken Pomodoro Farro Bowl, 99
  Seafood à la Paella with Farro, 111
Fats, 6–7, 13
Fish and seafood, 12
  Blackened Fish with Bean Salad, 104
  Caramelized Onions and Spinach with
    Glazed Balsamic Salmon, 87–88
  Fish Tacos with Mango and Kiwi Salsa, 84
  Fried Shrimp Brown Rice, 110
  Salmon Cakes Salad, 90–91
  Seafood à la Paella with Farro, 111
  Sheet Pan Glazed Balsamic Salmon
    with Asparagus, 105
  Shrimp and Vegetable Wild
    Rice Bowl, 100–101
Fried Shrimp Brown Rice, 110
Frittata, Sun-Dried Tomato and
  Vegetable, 64–65
Fruits, 11. *See also specific*
  Baked Mixed Fruit with Cinnamon, 144
  Dried Fruit and Chia High-
    Protein Muffins, 72–73
  Mixed Dried Fruit with
    Parmesan Cheese, 136

G

Glazed Pork Tenderloin and
  Bell Peppers, 130–131
Gluten-free
  Applesauce with Seeds, 138
  Baked Mixed Fruit with Cinnamon, 144
  Basic Brown Rice, 150
  Basic Flavorful Quinoa, 151
  Berry Mango Bliss Smoothie, 56
  Black Bean, Corn, and Chicken
    Sausage Bowl, 98

Blackened Fish with Bean Salad, 104
Cacao Coconut Cranberry Quinoa
  Breakfast Bowl, 61
California-Style Scrambled Eggs, 63
Caramelized Onions and Spinach with
  Glazed Balsamic Salmon, 87–88
Chia Cacao Pudding, 142
Chicken and Potato Salad with
  Yogurt Dressing, 92
Chicken Apple Salad, 82
Chicken Cilantro Patties, 89
Cilantro-Infused Yogurt Dressing, 156
Citrus Quinoa Avocado Salad
  with Roasted Chicken, 83
Creamy Green Smoothie, 57
Crustless Egg and Spinach Quiches, 66
Electric Pressure Cooker Red
  Lentil Soup, 126
Fish Tacos with Mango and
  Kiwi Salsa, 84
Glazed Pork Tenderloin and
  Bell Peppers, 130–131
Ground Turkey and Vegetable
  Stuffed Bell Peppers, 118–119
Hard-Boiled Egg and Apple Slices, 139
Lean Beef Meatballs in Tomato
  Sauce with Polenta, 128–129
Lemon-Mustard Vinaigrette, 155
Mango Lime Mousse, 145
Mason Jar Roasted Vegetable Soup
  with Parmesan Cheese, 140
Mini Parfait, 137
Mixed Berries Sweet Sauce, 158
Mixed Dried Fruit with
  Parmesan Cheese, 136
Orange Delight Smoothie, 55
Ricotta à la Méditerranée, 143
Roasted Chicken, 148
Roasted Vegetables, 154
Sheet Pan Glazed Balsamic Salmon
  with Asparagus, 105
Sheet Pan Mediterranean Chicken
  with Butternut Squash, 109
Steamed Broccoli and Cauliflower
  with Lemon Juice, 152–153

Sun-Dried Tomato and Vegetable
    Frittata, 64–65
Superfood Parfait, 58
Tomato Chickpea Soup, 93
Turkey Meatball Quinoa Soup, 94–95
Umami Scrambled Eggs, 62
Vegetable-Layered Cheese Lasagna, 127
Wild Fiesta Rice with Roasted Chicken, 115
Yellow Lentil Dip, 157
Yellow Lentil Dip with Olives
    and Red Peppers, 141
Goal-setting, 5–6
Ground Pork Endive Cups, 85
Ground Turkey and Vegetable
    Stuffed Bell Peppers, 118–119

H

Ham, Egg, and Cheese English
    Muffins, 68–69
Hard-Boiled Egg and Apple Slices, 139
High-intensity interval training (HIIT), 18
High-Protein Overnight Oats, 60
Hydration, 9

K

Kiwi and Mango Salsa, Fish Tacos with, 84

L

Lasagna, Vegetable-Layered Cheese, 127
Lean Beef Meatballs in Tomato
    Sauce with Polenta, 128–129
Legumes, 12
Lemons
    Lemon-Mustard Vinaigrette, 155
    Steamed Broccoli and Cauliflower
        with Lemon Juice, 152–153
Lentils
    Electric Pressure Cooker Red
        Lentil Soup, 126
    Yellow Lentil Dip, 157
    Yellow Lentil Dip with Olives
        and Red Peppers, 141
Light Farfalle and Cheese with
    Cauliflower, 96–97
Lime Mango Mousse, 145

Lower body exercises
    burpees, 23
    lunges, 22
    squats, 21

M

Mangos
    Baked Mixed Fruit with Cinnamon, 144
    Berry Mango Bliss Smoothie, 56
    Fish Tacos with Mango and Kiwi Salsa, 84
    Mango Lime Mousse, 145
Mason Jar Roasted Vegetable Soup
    with Parmesan Cheese, 140
Mayo-Yogurt Baked Chicken with
    Mini Potatoes, 116–117
Meal plans
    about, 33
    week 1, 34–37
    week 2, 38–41
    week 3, 42–45
    week 4, 46–49
Meatballs
    Lean Beef Meatballs in Tomato
        Sauce with Polenta, 128–129
    Turkey Meatball Quinoa Soup, 94–95
Meats, 12. *See also specific*
Mini Parfait, 137
Mixed Berries Sweet Sauce, 158
Mixed Dried Fruit with Parmesan
    Cheese, 136
Moody, Destini, 15
Mousse, Mango Lime, 145
Muffins, Dried Fruit and Chia
    High-Protein, 72–73
Mushrooms
    Electric Pressure Cooker Chicken,
        White Beans, Spinach, and
        Mushrooms in White Wine, 122–123
    Electric Pressure Cooker Low-Cal
        Beef Bourguignon, 124–125

N

Nutrient-dense foods, 6–7
Nuts, 13
    Butternut Squash Walnut Bread, 74–75

O

Oats
  Banana Cacao Oat Pancakes, 67
  High-Protein Overnight Oats, 60
  Spice-Infused Oatmeal, 59
Olives and Red Peppers, Yellow
    Lentil Dip with, 141
Onions
  Caramelized Onions and
      Spinach with Glazed Balsamic
      Salmon, 87–88
  Electric Pressure Cooker Low-Cal
      Beef Bourguignon, 124–125
Oranges
  Citrus Quinoa Avocado Salad
      with Roasted Chicken, 83
  Orange Delight Smoothie, 55

P

Pancakes, Banana Cacao Oat, 67
Panini, Roast Beef and Cheese, 79
Parfaits
  Mini Parfait, 137
  Superfood Parfait, 58
Parmesan cheese
  Mason Jar Roasted Vegetable
      Soup with Parmesan
      Cheese, 140
  Mixed Dried Fruit with
      Parmesan Cheese, 136
Pasta
  Light Farfalle and Cheese with
      Cauliflower, 96–97
  Pork Primavera Pasta, 132–133
Peruvian-Style Arroz con Pollo, 113–114
Pita Wraps, Curried Chicken, 81
Pizza, Sheet Pan Cracked-Egg, 108
Polenta, Lean Beef Meatballs in
    Tomato Sauce with, 128–129
Pork
  Glazed Pork Tenderloin and
      Bell Peppers, 130–131
  Ground Pork Endive Cups, 85
  Pork Primavera Pasta, 132–133

Portion sizes, 7
Potatoes
  Chicken and Potato Salad with
      Yogurt Dressing, 92
  Mayo-Yogurt Baked Chicken with
      Mini Potatoes, 116–117
Produce, 6, 11. See also specific
Proteins, 6, 9, 12
Pudding, Chia Cacao, 142

Q

Quiches, Crustless Egg and
    Spinach, 66
Quinoa
  Basic Flavorful Quinoa, 151
  Cacao Coconut Cranberry Quinoa
      Breakfast Bowl, 61
  Citrus Quinoa Avocado Salad
      with Roasted Chicken, 83
  Turkey Meatball Quinoa Soup, 94–95

R

Rice
  Basic Brown Rice, 150
  Fried Shrimp Brown Rice, 110
  Peruvian-Style Arroz con Pollo, 113–114
  Shrimp and Vegetable Wild
      Rice Bowl, 100–101
  Wild Fiesta Rice with Roasted
      Chicken, 115
Ricotta à la Méditerranée, 143
Roast Beef and Cheese Panini, 79
Roasted Chicken, 148
Roasted Vegetables, 154

S

Salads
  Blackened Fish with Bean Salad, 104
  Chicken and Potato Salad with
      Yogurt Dressing, 92
  Chicken Apple Salad, 82
  Citrus Quinoa Avocado Salad
      with Roasted Chicken, 83
  Ground Pork Endive Cups, 85
  Salmon Cakes Salad, 90–91

Salmon
  Caramelized Onions and Spinach with
    Glazed Balsamic Salmon, 87–88
  Salmon Cakes Salad, 90–91
  Sheet Pan Glazed Balsamic Salmon
    with Asparagus, 105
Salsa, Mango and Kiwi, Fish Tacos
  with, 84
Sandwiches. *See also* Wraps
  Avocado, Tomato, and Poached
    Egg Toast, 78
  Egg, Cheese, and Ham English
    Muffins, 68–69
  Roast Beef and Cheese Panini, 79
Seafood à la Paella with Farro, 111
Seeds, 13
  Applesauce with Seeds, 138
  Chia Cacao Pudding, 142
  Dried Fruit and Chia High-
    Protein Muffins, 72–73
Sheet Pan Cracked-Egg
  Pizza, 108
Sheet Pan Glazed Balsamic Salmon
  with Asparagus, 105
Sheet Pan Mediterranean Chicken
  with Butternut Squash, 109
Sheet Pan Roasted Tofu and
  Cauliflower, 106–107
Shrimp
  Fried Shrimp Brown Rice, 110
  Seafood à la Paella with Farro, 111
  Shrimp and Vegetable Wild
    Rice Bowl, 100–101
SMART goals, 5–6
Smoothies
  Berry Mango Bliss Smoothie, 56
  Creamy Green Smoothie, 57
  Orange Delight Smoothie, 55
  Warm Apple-Spiced Smoothie, 54
Snacks, 9
  Applesauce with Seeds, 138
  Hard-Boiled Egg and Apple Slices, 139
  Mason Jar Roasted Vegetable Soup
    with Parmesan Cheese, 140
  Mini Parfait, 137

  Mixed Dried Fruit with
    Parmesan Cheese, 136
  Yellow Lentil Dip with Olives
    and Red Peppers, 141
Soups and stews
  Chicken Pomodoro Farro Bowl, 99
  Electric Pressure Cooker Red
    Lentil Soup, 126
  Mason Jar Roasted Vegetable Soup
    with Parmesan Cheese, 140
  Tomato Chickpea Soup, 93
  Turkey Meatball Quinoa Soup, 94–95
Spice-Infused Oatmeal, 59
Spinach
  Caramelized Onions and Spinach with
    Glazed Balsamic Salmon, 87–88
  Creamy Green Smoothie, 57
  Crustless Egg and Spinach Quiches, 66
  Electric Pressure Cooker Chicken,
    White Beans, Spinach, and
    Mushrooms in White Wine, 122–123
  Turkey Spinach Roll, 80
Steamed Broccoli and Cauliflower
  with Lemon Juice, 152–153
Stir-fries
  Beef and Vegetable Stir-Fry, 121
  Chickpea Stir-Fry, 120
  Shrimp and Vegetable Wild
    Rice Bowl, 100–101
Strength/resistance training, 18
Sun-Dried Tomato and Vegetable
  Frittata, 64–65
Superfood Parfait, 58

T

Tacos, Fish, with Mango and Kiwi Salsa, 84
"Talk to Your Hand" rule, 7
Toast, Avocado, Tomato, and
  Poached Egg, 78
Tofu and Cauliflower, Sheet Pan
  Roasted, 106–107
Tomatoes
  Avocado, Tomato, and Poached
    Egg Toast, 78
  Chicken Pomodoro Farro Bowl, 99

Tomatoes (*continued*)
  Lean Beef Meatballs in Tomato
    Sauce with Polenta, 128–129
  Sun-Dried Tomato and Vegetable
    Frittata, 64–65
  Tomato Chickpea Soup, 93
Turkey
  Ground Turkey and Vegetable
    Stuffed Bell Peppers, 118–119
  Turkey Meatball Quinoa Soup, 94–95
  Turkey Spinach Roll, 80

U

Umami Scrambled Eggs, 62
Upper body exercises
  biceps curls, 27
  push-ups, 24–25
  triceps dips, 26

V

Vegan
  Applesauce with Seeds, 138
  Baked Mixed Fruit with Cinnamon, 144
  Chickpea Stir-Fry, 120
  Electric Pressure Cooker Red
    Lentil Soup, 126
  Lemon-Mustard Vinaigrette, 155
  Mixed Berries Sweet Sauce, 158
  Roasted Vegetables, 154
  Sheet Pan Roasted Tofu and
    Cauliflower, 106–107
  Steamed Broccoli and Cauliflower
    with Lemon Juice, 152–153
  Yellow Lentil Dip, 157
  Yellow Lentil Dip with Olives
    and Red Peppers, 141
Vegetables, 9, 11. *See also specific*
  Beef and Vegetable Stir-Fry, 121
  Ground Turkey and Vegetable
    Stuffed Bell Peppers, 118–119
  Mason Jar Roasted Vegetable Soup
    with Parmesan Cheese, 140
  Roasted Vegetables, 154
  Shrimp and Vegetable Wild
    Rice Bowl, 100–101

Sun-Dried Tomato and Vegetable
  Frittata, 64–65
Vegetable-Layered Cheese Lasagna, 127
Vegetarian. *See also* Vegan
  Avocado, Tomato, and Poached
    Egg Toast, 78
  Banana Cacao Oat Pancakes, 67
  Berry Mango Bliss Smoothie, 56
  Butternut Squash Walnut Bread, 74–75
  Cacao Coconut Cranberry Quinoa
    Breakfast Bowl, 61
  California-Style Scrambled Eggs, 63
  Chia Cacao Pudding, 142
  Cilantro-Infused Yogurt Dressing, 156
  Creamy Green Smoothie, 57
  Crustless Egg and Spinach Quiches, 66
  Dried Fruit and Chia High-
    Protein Muffins, 72–73
  Egg and Avocado Burritos, 70–71
  Hard-Boiled Egg and Apple Slices, 139
  High-Protein Overnight Oats, 60
  Light Farfalle and Cheese with
    Cauliflower, 96–97
  Mango Lime Mousse, 145
  Mini Parfait, 137
  Mixed Dried Fruit with
    Parmesan Cheese, 136
  Orange Delight Smoothie, 55
  Ricotta à la Méditerranée, 143
  Sheet Pan Cracked-Egg Pizza, 108
  Spice-Infused Oatmeal, 59
  Sun-Dried Tomato and Vegetable
    Frittata, 64–65
  Superfood Parfait, 58
  Umami Scrambled Eggs, 62
  Vegetable-Layered Cheese Lasagna, 127
  Warm Apple-Spiced Smoothie, 54

W

Walnut Butternut Squash Bread, 74–75
Warm Apple-Spiced Smoothie, 54
White Wine, Electric Pressure Cooker
  Chicken, White Beans, Spinach,
  and Mushrooms in, 122–123
Whole grains, 7, 12

Wild Fiesta Rice with Roasted Chicken, 115
Workout plan, 31
Wraps
  Curried Chicken Pita Wraps, 81
  Egg and Avocado Burritos, 70–71
  Fish Tacos with Mango and Kiwi Salsa, 84
  Turkey Spinach Roll, 80

Y
Yellow Lentil Dip, 157
Yellow Lentil Dip with Olives
    and Red Peppers, 141

Yogurt
  Chicken and Potato Salad with
      Yogurt Dressing, 92
  Cilantro-Infused Yogurt Dressing, 156
  High-Protein Overnight Oats, 60
  Mayo-Yogurt Baked Chicken with
      Mini Potatoes, 116–117
  Mini Parfait, 137
  Superfood Parfait, 58

Acknowledgments

I want to thank Destini Moody for her writing contributions, and Alejandro Pinot for recipe development assistance.

About the Author

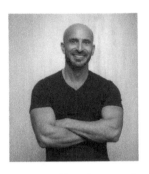 **Manuel Villacorta, MS, RDN,** is an internationally recognized, award-winning registered dietitian-nutritionist with more than 18 years of experience. He is a bestselling author and has published five additional books.

Manuel is one of the leading weight loss and nutrition experts in the country and the recipient of five "Best Bay Area Nutritionist" awards from the *San Francisco Chronicle* and ABC7 News. He was named the "2019 Influencer of the Year" by the Produce for Better Health Foundation.

Manuel is a respected and trusted voice in the health and wellness industry. His knowledge, charismatic talent, and English/Spanish bilingual proficiency have made him an in-demand health and nutrition expert on national and international television.

Born and raised in Peru, Manuel currently lives in San Francisco, California. He earned his BS in nutrition and physiology metabolism from the University of California, Berkeley, and his MS in nutrition and food science from California State University, San Jose.